Dukan Diet 2
The 7 Steps

Dr Pierre Dukan

Dukan Diet 2
The 7 Steps

HODDER &
STOUGHTON

First published as *Léscalier Nutrionnel* in France in 2014 by J'ai Lu Librio

First published in Great Britain in 2015 by Hodder & Stoughton
An Hachette UK company

1

A CIP catalogue record for this title is available from the British Library

Trade paperback ISBN 978 1 473 60994 5
Ebook ISBN 978 1 473 60995 2

Typeset in Celeste by Hewer Text UK Ltd, Edinburgh

Printed and bound by Clays Ltd, St Ives plc

Hodder & Stoughton policy is to use papers that are natural, renewable
and recyclable products and made from wood grown in sustainable
forests. The logging and manufacturing processes are expected to
conform to the environmental regulations of the country of origin.

Hodder & Stoughton Ltd
338 Euston Road
London NW1 3BH

www.hodder.co.uk

Contents

III. FIGHTING AT YOUR SIDE

CONCLUSION   395

Introduction

THIS IS A COMMITTED AND PROACTIVE BOOK, FULL OF FIRE AND PASSION

This is also a book of war, because when it comes to weight problems we're facing an unforgiving enemy. And I know this enemy well; as a doctor and nutritionist, my work has been devoted to tracking it down. Its strength lies in the way it cleverly insinuates itself into our lives under the friendly guise of *bon viveur* and enjoyment of the good things life has to offer. But let's face the facts: for millions around the world this stealthy adversary is gaining the upper hand. In France alone, there are 27 million overweight people, of whom 7 million are obese, trapped and vulnerable. They're also vaguely aware, without taking it fully on board, that their lives will be nine years shorter than other people's.

Perhaps you know my method and the diet named after me. Its success turned my life upside down and radically changed my reasons for living. This all began for me at an age when most people are thinking about their retirement. Today, I realize that I'm getting involved in the midst of a battle – one that certainly fires you with enthusiasm, but one that is also terribly unequal. This is a battle between the individual and a disease of civilization, a pandemic, the first avoidable plague to beset the human race. Mindful of this power struggle, I feel compelled more than ever by the urgent need to strive to do better, to be inventive and innovative, so as to hone my weapons and retaliate with even greater strength.

And this is the reason why, given the current world-wide weight problem crisis, I'm opening up a second line of attack, **a second front**, on the battleground.

Although very different from the first front, the second adheres to its values and philosophy. It can therefore work alongside my original method to reach a wider audience, to bring on board and offer help to a different section of the population.

I know that the Dukan Diet is well known for being both extremely effective and strict. It is also very demanding, suiting the most determined dieters.

Over recent years, I've come to realize that there are also overweight people out there who are in less of a hurry to lose weight. They have moderate weight problems, a less compulsive appetite, a very busy and open social life and have less of a medical risk. They feel less inclined to go for a long time without enjoying a tasty treat, a glass of wine or a few squares of chocolate. In a nutshell, there are people whose motivation hasn't yet reached its peak but **who want to lose weight**

nevertheless, well aware that their weight problems could well escalate.

I am myself well aware that some of these people got caught up in the general excitement of the previous decade, tried my diet but struggled with its rigorousness, and so didn't manage to continue right to the end.

It's for anyone who can't see themselves following my original method that I devised, practised and tested the Nutritional Staircase, my second front.

So from now on, there isn't just a single way of tackling weight problems with my help but two: the first one, which some people have described as 'the strong way', and the second, 'the gentle way'. This book explains how to use it and everything you need to know so that you can choose *your* path and *your* solution from these two strategies.

My work as a practitioner, with patients whom I treated in traditional personal consultations, convinced me that it was possible to fight weight problems and get results. I started my career very early on and, for well over 40 years, I've helped and supported a great number of patients. During the first 30 years, dissatisfied with what I'd learnt while specializing in nutrition, I took the liberty of breaking out of the mould to invent and patiently shape my own method. As time went by, I was so convinced by its results and effectiveness that I felt the need to reach a wider audience by promoting the method in a book for the general public. *Je ne sais pas maigrir* (the original French version of the Dukan Diet) was published in 2000, and was amazingly successful. It has been read in over 50 countries by almost 35 million people, including 16 million in France. The diet associated with it has had a massive following. I say this without wishing to sound boastful or flatter my own ego, but rather to show the extent to which the book and method inspired hope.

Recently, I was most impatient and eager to see the results of the ObEpi study published by a French institution which brings out a report every three years on how weight issues affect the French population. In 2013, the ObEpi study revealed – and for the first time since it has been collecting such data – that between 2009 and 2012, the period during which my influence and work as a nutritionist were at their height in France, there had been an extreme **decrease** in the phenomenon of weight problems and obesity.

Among the population spared the increase in weight problems were obese people, of whom one-third (i.e. about 500,000) were over 55 (according to the 2009 survey). They belonged to that section of the French population at greatest risk of morbidity and mortality. As a doctor, I know that a large section of this at-risk population adjusted the course of their lives and, probably without realizing it, escaped the cruel clutches of a tragic fate.

Furthermore, an obesity study, supervised by the Department of Nutrition at the Pitié-Salpêtrière

Hospital in Paris, examined the effectiveness of the Dukan method's Stabilization phase. Here are the results: of 4,500 women who had lost weight, 36 per cent had not regained any two years later; and after five years, 20 per cent were deemed to be 'cured' of their weight problems. Compared with the 3 per cent who are cured worldwide when all diets are taken into account, this is a fantastic result. It's quite unheard of and amazingly encouraging – an extra 17 per cent!

So yes, I am indeed writing a book of war, and if I run the risk of appearing immodest, it's so that you understand that the issues at stake are of great importance to YOU and this is why I need to convince you.

The truth I've arrived at, which I've learnt through my career as a campaigning doctor and nutritionist, is that the war against weight problems, with all the death and suffering it causes, is a war that nobody wants to wage and even less one that anyone wants to win.

Given what appears in the media and the number of decision-makers we hear moaning and getting worked up about the extent of the threat, this may seem surprising to you. However, there is a very simple explanation. Our globalized world is governed by the market economy, of this you will be aware. So what does the logic of the market say? That if this war was properly waged and won, if a method could help all these individuals lose weight, then part of the food-processing industry, the part that promotes and supplies snack products, and part of the pharmaceutical industry, the part that treats repercussions from weight problems, would be damaged. We know full well that, in many countries, and certainly in France, both industries figure among the most powerful and profitable.

The market is pragmatic. It readily admits that if weight issues were controlled, the public health budget would stand to gain a great deal. But it also states just as clearly that the national economy would lose infinitely more were this to happen. This is the unfortunate truth. However, everyone has to choose between the need for their society's economic growth and what they need for their personal existence, their individual well-being, their quality of life, their image, their relationship with others and themselves, their self-esteem and, lastly, their health and even their life.

I'll say it again, it may seem like we're hitting against an insurmountable wall, UNLESS out of this conflict between society's economic health and the health of individuals a new force can be brought to life that fully benefits both. Coca-Cola, for example, has developed soft drinks, Diet Coke and Coke Zero, for people watching their weight. Rather than making money from a drink known to have played a major role in the explosion of American obesity, Coca-Cola has instead managed to invent an alternative, without any sugar or glucose syrup, which today earns the company enormous profits. Many other manufacturers are following suit, including those who make cereal-based products, and selling low-sugar, low-fat versions of their products without additives and colourings.

I am campaigning fervently for an economy to emerge that grows richer from the fight against weight issues rather than one that makes money out of contributing to weight problems.

I'll go much further: for years I've been campaigning for France to become the leading country in the struggle against weight problems, an international laboratory that would develop beneficial suggestions to help the one and a half billion people across the world who are overweight or obese.

Because France is without doubt the one country that has the greatest legitimacy to a say in this fight. France's culture of gastronomy has been added to UNESCO's Intangible World Heritage List; we also have many great international chefs and a whole range of wonderful local products. French women are famous for their slim figures and elegance. Our luxury goods, haute couture and tourism industries are world renowned. I have no doubt that French opinion would be listened to and widely followed across the planet.

The change from treating my patients directly and personally to treating them indirectly through my books made me realize just how useful this second front can be.

For a long time now, I've been convinced that weight problems in France and elsewhere are spreading at such a rate that the traditional solution of one-to-one medical consultations can no longer contain them.

There are, of course, still a few patients who can find a nutritionist to supervise their weight-loss programme, but there will never be enough health professionals to look after 27 million overweight people! Only a mass media can have any chance of success when it comes to tackling a disease of civilization on such a scale. That was why, back in 2000, I wrote my first book, without ever imagining that it would reach such a wide readership. When I saw this happen, I stopped my daily dozen or so patient consultations so that I could help the tens of millions of other people from all over the world.

Nonetheless, losing weight with a book as your only guide and support requires a certain determination and motivation, particular needs, and a character and psychological profile that not everyone possesses.

It was when I realized that my initial method might be too combative, too demanding and for some even too quick that I endeavoured to come up with an entirely new approach, so that these people wouldn't get lost en route. Over a long period, I tested this Nutritional Staircase to see how useful, effective and well-received it would be. Today, this new method is fully ready and has been honed down to the very last details. I intend to make use of it to stand up to the current 'down with diets' trend, an opportunist fad that has come over from the States and which reappears from time to time whenever diets are gaining ground and threatening the market.

This trend is not only useless, it is actually dangerous, since it aims to de-motivate anyone reluctant to give up the comfort they get from eating, which helps them cope with stress and adversity.

In France, for example, obese men and women over 55 with diabetes or high blood pressure are dying prematurely on a daily basis. Some of them would still be alive today if they hadn't been put off losing weight through dieting.

Currently, dieting is the only way we know of to reduce surplus weight as well as diabetes, high blood pressure and the various risks connected with 'diabesity'.

Entirely dreamt up by American psychologists, the diet backlash is based on two fallacious arguments:

• **The first argument** is that modern man is incapable of making the effort to follow a diet. This effort would be so traumatic that after slimming down modern man would put the weight back on and could even end up suffering from eating disorders. French supporters of this American trend – which one might suspect is not unconnected to the chocolate, sugar and flour industry, given the extent to which its interests are served – sing the same chorus, that my method is too frustrating and too hard to follow.

It is not frustrating, first and foremost because the results are obvious and quick to appear, and moreover because anyone following this diet can eat 100 foods and eat as much of them as they want. As for all other foods, you are allowed to eat them in a selective, gradual and carefully planned way.

Many people who've lost weight with my method can testify to how easy it was for them to follow. So great and rewarding was the happiness of successfully dieting that the unavoidable changes that my programme suggests for shedding these annoying, even handicapping pounds, were accepted. My patients could enjoy looking at themselves in the mirror, be delighted at getting back their old figure and most importantly rediscovering their self-confidence and *joie de vivre*. Many of them use the same expression to unambiguously voice their satisfaction: 'It has changed my life!' I can recall one woman telling me: 'When I lose weight this way, I get more pleasure from slimming than from eating comfort food.' My original method is not difficult to follow; it is simple, strict and coherent.

- **The second argument** of the 'down with diets' brigade is that they're dangerous. My answer to this is that not only is it untrue, but when we consider just how extremely damaging obesity and weight problems are, what is actually dangerous is for an effective diet to be unavailable or refused. It's obvious that if a person has put on weight and a lot of it, food and excessive eating signal a vulnerability, and their comfort eating is a way of coping with their vulnerability. Who hasn't tried to assuage their anger or soothe their sorrow through eating? But for some people this is systematic, which is where the danger lies for their health. That said, I'm amazed that what is so glaringly obvious and common-sensical has to be proved. Losing weight and shifting your surplus pounds means you're getting rid of a handicap and an unnecessary burden; losing weight can only improve health; it reduces blood sugar levels; it lowers blood pressure, thus alleviating the direct threat posed to the brain and heart by hypertension. Losing weight lightens the load carried by the vertebral joints, the hips and knees, and it almost systematically puts a stop to sleep apnoeas, which spoil your life and can end up endangering it. Cutting down your weight is as life-saving as stopping smoking or giving up the bottle if you're an alcoholic. However, such is the economic weight of the food-processing lobbies, and their sphere of influence so great and so widespread, that the case for the health benefits of weight-loss dieting has to be made tirelessly in order for the idea to be accepted.

THIS BOOK IS THEREFORE ABOUT OPENING UP A SECOND FRONT IN THE WAR AGAINST WEIGHT PROBLEMS

Why this second front and what does it offer?

As I've already outlined, my first front is the method I devised between 1970 and 2000, a diet that people who used it named after me. For the first six years after *Je ne sais pas maigrir* was published, my method operated far from the spotlight. It was passed on simply by word of mouth and then mainly on the great communication hub of the internet. Those who had success with it said so in their own way, with their own words, and with a sincere desire to pass the message on. After these six years, the global bookstore Amazon sent out a press release stating that sales of my book had outstripped those of *Harry Potter*.

Totally unknown to the press and the media at the time, I remember the day when this was announced because no fewer than 17 journalists called me, wanting to know who I was. During the next six years, this book maintained its popularity and I went on to write other books which, like the first, travelled worldwide to spread the message that a – French – method was helping people lose weight and doing better than anything else that had gone before. I gradually came to realise that weight problems and obesity, which are now seen everywhere as a modern pandemic of mankind, were perhaps not an inescapable fact of life; it was possible to slow down the growth of weight problems and have the ambitious goal of driving them back and putting an end to them. One and a half billion overweight people, with a third of them obese, were not unavoidably condemned to stay this way.

The enormous wave of enthusiasm for my diet ruffled quite a few feathers. A great number of small and large vested interests felt threatened by my work and ganged up against it. This gave me lots to ponder, with humility and a constructive mind. What I had learnt from my patients over a fairly long period as a practitioner was how they can think and act without always being totally aware or fully in control. By drawing on my feelings and my empathy, I was finally able to immerse myself in their psychology. Whenever a man or woman puts on weight, it never happens because they intended it to happen.

Once the weight gain gets too much, it causes dissatisfaction then misery, but it still doesn't stop the underlying behaviour causing it. Why and how can a 5ft 5in woman, who weighed just over 10 stone after having her first child at 25, let herself put on another stone and a half by the time she's 30, while being alarmed about this – and then creep up to 13 or even 14 stone a few years later? I have seen this many times in my consultations.

If the man or woman who puts on weight is tolerating such agony then it's because they're coping with some other far more intense agony. Agony that is hidden or difficult to discern, which they try to cancel out with a natural pleasure that they use excessively or compulsively.

And then the time comes when this weight gain becomes overwhelming and more difficult to bear than the underlying misery that caused it. The cup is full and the decision to slim down becomes inevitable, just like a ripe fruit that comes away from the branch.

Given the emotional profile of people who've grown fat by using food as a crutch, the question now is: how are they going to manage without it and what could possibly replace it?

The answer my method – the first front – gave was that the best reward lies in the very success of dieting: shedding those pounds and rediscovering your self-esteem. For this to happen from the word go, I tried to give my patients a weight-loss plan that above all worked very well, especially right at the beginning to boost motivation. For people who didn't think themselves capable, losing a lot of weight and quickly is a very powerful reason to feel proud and a sense of self-worth. The immediate joy of losing weight anaesthetizes the potential difficulty of doing it.

However, amid the biased, partisan attacks unleashed by the success of my method, I also heard touching messages from people who had given up partway because they were hypersensitive, vulnerable and, most especially, influenced by the prevailing 'down with diets' attitude. I was touched by their messages and I **asked myself whether the strictness that suited some so well might not put others off, leaving them by the wayside** and willing to give credence to the dream merchants advocating that we abandon dieting.

I also heard all those people who, having lost weight with my diet, had put it back on because they didn't follow the last two phases and were unsure if they'd be able to give it another try with as much enthusiasm and motivation as before.

Lastly, I heard those people who didn't feel ready or sufficiently overweight to get involved with such a head-on approach. People who weren't in a hurry or troubled by some worrying pathology, or who quite simply lacked the heroic fibre and felt the very human need to give in to temptation, unable to imagine a couple of months without a glass of wine or nibbling a few squares of chocolate, or enjoying a meal with friends in a restaurant at the weekend, but who nonetheless wanted to slim down.

According to my personal statistics, collected using a questionnaire inserted into my books, half of my readers managed to lose weight and half of those then managed to stabilize. **So I'm aiming this second front partly at anyone who failed to lose weight or was unable to stabilize or whose motivation wasn't quite at its peak.**

I've always been, and still am, very much in contact with the many people who get in touch with me. Some patients, who've failed with their attempt, ask me if they can go back to the initial method, the first front, and start again from scratch. They want to throw themselves back into the fray, ready to take up arms once more and return to the battlefield knowing where they went wrong, more determined than ever to succeed. And I know that they'll do it, because they're motivated and inspired by the challenge, the confrontation and success.

A diet doesn't always achieve its objective the first time round. Both experience and my statistics show that dieters who reprise the original method in this way do indeed succeed, like those smokers who often find that they manage to give up on their second attempt.

However, it was the other dieters who spoke to me, those for whom the original version of my method was too ambitious or seemed too harsh because of where they were then at in their lives. A person may well no longer feel able today to follow the same diet they were quite happy trying yesterday.

And then I thought about those people who demand too much from comfort eating to be able to give it up entirely for several days, and those who have too little to lose to want to try such an effective diet or who are more epicurean than stoic.

So it's for them that I am now opening up this second front – so that I can win them over and, most importantly, not abandon them to the power of the lobbies and the supporters of such lobbies, whether intentional or not.

Finally, I'd like to thank Dr Atkins and Dr Montignac (who died in 2010), whom I managed to meet in New York and Paris respectively. Both talented nutritionists, they told me about their careers and their fight against obesity and weight problems. I learnt much from what they told me and from their difficulties in getting a different approach to dieting accepted. It's a shame that they didn't write about their own story and research, as I'm convinced that they've both made important contributions to innovating twentieth-century nutrition.

I

THE FIRST FRONT

or

'The Strong Way'

The War Against Weight Problems

I've used the term 'front' to place myself straightaway in a battle context. This is a cause made legitimate by the ravaging effects of weight problems, ranked by the World Health Organization (WHO) as the fifth most serious scourge afflicting mankind. I'm positioning myself as a combatant.

As I've said, nowadays nobody gets fat intentionally. If over time you've gained some weight, pound after pound, sometimes stone after stone, obviously you were not a willing party. It may be that members of your family tend to put on weight. The influence of genetic factors cannot be denied, but it's only part of the story and it certainly isn't decisive. It may be that in early childhood your emotional development was so disturbed that it created an 'oral' vulnerability in you. Psychologists refer to this as 'flight to food', triggered by hypersensitivity to your environment and an inability to tolerate stress. However, even if we put these two factors together, in no way do they explain why there are one and a half billion people in the world with weight problems.

I can explain it by what I call the 'happiness disease'. As we make our way in the world, as we are moulded and shaped, a growing number of us fail to find happiness. If I state this so abruptly, it's for the simple reason that I'm conscious of saying something scandalous. When half the adult population of a country like France, for example, is well and truly overweight, and a great many people are suffering from feeling imprisoned in an unloved and unhealthy body, it's time to stop blaming it on trivial, personal and random reasons or on a lack of willpower. What we need is a more comprehensive explanation.

My opinion, based on observing thousands of patients and my experience of analyzing cases over a long career, is that becoming overweight has far more to do with society and behaviour than with nutrition. We should just remember *two decisive facts*:

1. Did you know that being overweight is an extremely recent phenomenon and before 1944 simply did not exist for any composite population group, *nor was it even recorded?* Today, this phenomenon is found in any nation anywhere in the world, except in those countries where famine reigns.
2. The phenomenon of obesity is most prevalent in the United States, the country that invented and spread the new way of life in which we're steeped.

The cause of this phenomenon has to be structural for it to have invaded the entire world to such an extent and in such a short space of time. What gives it away is that in 1944 we moved into a world governed by market forces. And, since the prevalence of the economy is now the order of things, we have to accept it. But individuals must have the opportunity to defend and protect themselves and keep their children away from it. To do this, you need to have enough of the right information at your fingertips, so that you can decide your own destiny and future.

This being the case, whenever I talk about battles and am taken to task for using warlike language, it's because people want to conceal the danger, the threat that for over half a century has been spreading like an oil slick across the planet. China, which only 15 years ago was spared the danger of weight problems, is now in absolute terms the country with the greatest overweight population in the world. And, what is far more serious, it has the greatest prevalence of infantile diabetes, a condition that didn't even exist when I was a medical student.

For decades, we were 'playing for time', as we considered any concern to control weight as just a notion or a whim that preoccupied the fair sex. When we looked at an excessively fat person, we tended to see only the jolly outer appearance of a '*bon viveur*'. Whether intentionally or not, we played down weight issues; we underestimated the health problems caused by being overweight. We failed to warn people who were oblivious to the risks they were exposing themselves to as they carried on gaining weight.

Obesity is not an autonomous medical state. A person is not born into the world obese; they become obese. And it always starts off with being overweight, then, without even realizing it, once your BMI (Body Mass Index) rises from 29 to 30, you become obese. At that point, people deemed as rather too fond of their food are suddenly no longer *bon viveurs* but they now find themselves in the sphere of 'proper' medicine, with its cancer, diabetes and cardiovascular diseases. Encouraged to become over-weight and obese by corporations that sell 'violent' sugars – fast-acting carbs that cause the most damage – they are then treated and cared for by the corporations that sell medication.

From 1980 through to 1995, there was a regular and unstoppable increase in the numbers of people becom-ing overweight and obese. After the ban on appetite suppressants in 1997, the numbers soared and it became apparent that so-called traditional low-calorie diets had proved to be terribly ineffective. In the meantime, in parallel, the food-processing sector based on sugar, white flour and starchy foods saw its profits rise. This was mirrored in the pharmaceutical sector, which was selling medication to deal with the complications and comorbidities arising from these weight problems. This all had an extremely favourable impact on economic activity and, therefore, national wealth. It's probably the reason why anyone working in an area involved with the upsurge in weight problems is treated with indulgence.To take just one example from many, did you know that, in France, there is an annual Week of Taste (*semaine du goût*)? It has worked its way into nursery schools, where children are 'educated' to be fond of food, at an age when they are most impressionable as far as their emotions and senses are concerned. And who do you think sponsors this event? The sugar industry!

Since we can't change the world and its economic governance, the medical profession, manufacturers and politicians need to realize that they must mediate between the citizen and the state, between the economy and health. This is the where the future is heading, the path is wide open.

To have a clearer understanding of my second front so that you can follow it more easily, I think it's vital that I summarize the key principles of my original slimming method.

For years I worked in my surgery, fighting obesity and developing this method.

It involved a great deal of meticulous research to ensure that it really was effective. This method has meant that I've been able to draw on extraordinary support from an enthusiastic community of men and women who are proud of having succeeded in dealing with their problem. Living in all four corners of the world, in very diverse cultures with different eating habits, they turned to this method to lose weight and keep it off for good.

They've managed to do this, so you can manage to do it too. I'm convinced that this is what you want and need.

Please be aware that by opening up a second front, I've no intention whatsoever of replacing the first one. My second front is an extra front, to be added to the first.

If after reading this Nutritional Staircase you feel in more of a hurry to do battle with your extra pounds, then the first front would suit you better, at least for the time being. All you need do is refer to *The Dukan Diet*, where all my advice about how to proceed is explained in detail. Remember that my original method, the strong way, has a four-phase progression: two phases for losing weight very quickly – the speed is highly motivating and will help you attain your True Weight (which can be calculated for free on my website www.regimedukan.com) – followed by two phases to stop you ever putting any weight back on. The method extends over one, two or even three months, depending on how much you have to lose. With hindsight I can now see that it is similar to my own way of being: passionate, wholehearted, all or nothing, and only giving of my very best. And also that it suits a certain type of patient, those who fit this same mould. They've found that this method gave them not only a quick reward but enough of a reward all round to replace the comfort and gratification they had sought from fattening foods. And their success is what has most spurred me on to keep innovating.

You'll find the essential elements of my original method in the instructions and advice that make up the second front; however, this is arranged very differently. You organize your meals over a seven-day period, which is repeated over and over until your extra half-stone or one or two stone have disappeared. Thereafter, the guidelines for the (two-part) Consolidation phase and the Stabilization phase are the same as for the so-called strong way.

What Are the Initial Method's Key Points?

First and foremost, I gave up counting calories and all those low-calorie diets that don't work, opting instead for animal and plant (tempeh, tofu, seitan) proteins and vegetables. I discovered how useful oat bran is and konjac, which has no calories. At the same time, I thought long and hard about human nature and the 'happy' activities that are so often missing from the lives of people who are overweight or obese. I then worked out how long the four phases should last (Attack, Cruise, Consolidation and Stabilization). There was nothing at the time for the post-diet period – so I prescribed a long-term, balanced diet and advocated three simple measures that you follow for the rest of your life.

To sum up, here are the method's main features; you'll find the same features in the second front's method, too.

It's Simple

100 as-much-as-you-want foods: 72 protein foods – lean meat, veal, beef (except rib roast), offal; all fish and shell-fish; poultry without the skin, except duck and goose; low-fat cooked, sliced ham, turkey, chicken and pork;

eggs; vegetable proteins (tempeh, tofu, seitan, soya steaks); fat-free dairy products, yoghurts and cottage cheese.

And 28 vegetables (tomatoes, cucumber, radish, spinach, asparagus, leeks, green beans, cabbage, mushrooms, celery, fennel, lettuce, chicory, aubergines, courgettes, peppers, chard, and so on).

It's Natural

Since the beginnings of mankind up until 1944, the human diet consisted essentially of vegetables and proteins. They have been, and still are today, vital and beneficial for our bodies and our health.

It's Easy

You can eat until you feel satisfied, because you are allowed to eat the foodstuffs prescribed without any restriction on quantity. You're free to combine the foods as you wish and to eat whenever you fancy. This is both practical and gratifying. You can enjoy the pleasure of eating tasty, varied food and lots of it – you're strongly advised to use spices and condiments!

It's Strict

I've set up a strong structure to steer you. It's made up of four phases which follow on from one another so that you're looked after and guided as much as possible. It was important to me to find the very best way of supporting and encouraging you.

It Lasts

Protecting the weight you slim down to is hugely important, so two of the method's four phases are devoted to consolidating this weight and stabilizing it for the rest of your life. A wager, a challenge, and the proof that it is possible – you don't have to be overweight.

It's Varied

It comprises 2,000 amazing but simple recipes that come from all over the world. Tasty, original, but in keeping with the diet's nutritional programme, because if you've got to slim down you might as well do so with pleasure and enjoyment!

It's Innovative

I added oat bran to my eating programme making it part of the foundation. Oat bran has so many health-giving benefits which make it a vital ally – and it gets results.

It's Sensible

Your daily physical exercise focuses on walking; the prescribed dose is a 20-minute walk each day.

It's Convivial

Coaching and support have been developed to offer interactive personalized coaching via the internet. The coach provides instructions in the morning and the user then reports back in the evening. This system boosts motivation and strengthens your good intentions day by day.

It's Successful

And this, of course, is fundamental. Due to its effectiveness and the speed with which results are obtained, my method has been used by tens of millions of people who have passed the message on to others spontaneously. As far as I'm aware, my method has never caused the slightest harm to anyone.

If you're interested in the theory then, as far as metabolism is concerned, the way my method works is based on five points:

1. **It breaks with the system of counting calories** as it is still practised. This daily calorie-counting is based on a simple argument, one that seems obvious but which is nonetheless wrong. Calories serve as a unit of measurement and, by definition, one calorie is equivalent to another calorie, just like one gram is one gram. This is true if we take an abstract, theoretical calorie outside the body. However, calories only exist *inside* our bodies. And then the impact varies. I'll give you an example to show you what I mean. One pound is the same as another pound. We agree. Now imagine me throwing a pound of feathers out of a window followed by another pound but this time of lead. A passerby would much prefer to have the feathers fall on their head than the lead!

It's exactly the same for the calories the body takes from the different foods we give it; they are not all processed in the same way and do not affect the body in the same way.

The body digests and assimilates foods very differently according to their physical and chemical composition. This means that the body needs to make only a very small effort to break up 100 calories of sugar or oil so they can pass into the bloodstream. This process uses up only two or three calories. However, to break up the proteins in a steak into its amino acids and to get them into the blood one by one, the body will need to expend ten times more energy, i.e. 32 calories.

Furthermore, these calories come from foods with a very different taste, texture and consistency. We don't eat 100 calories of leeks or mussels in the same way or with quite the same enthusiasm as 100 calories of chocolate. The sensations are different and our brain can quite quickly get us to prefer chocolate to steamed leeks.

What is far, far worse is that as soon as sugars (fast carbs) get into the bloodstream, they trigger a defence reflex and insulin is secreted. This insulin then turns the sugar into fat and stores it away in our adipose tissue.

No, quite definitely, calories are not all much of a muchness.

2. **It points the finger at invasive, violent and fast carbs** as being primarily responsible for weight

problems, obesity and diabetes, encapsulated in the term 'diabesity'.

Glucose and fructose syrups, sugary fizzy drinks, refined white flours, white bread, corn flakes, sugars, sugary starchy foods, biscuit products and so on. Why are they dangerous? They have a quick, invasive penetration level – the glycaemic index – and, once inside the body, they're aggressive to the pancreas, which secretes insulin to protect us. The insulin drives back these carbs, turning them into fat, which gets stored away in the adipose tissue. As the years go by, the pancreas grows tired, cutting down its insulin production, and this leads to the onset of diabetes. Man's *physiology* cannot deal with the invasion of violent carbs without suffering damage. For the most part, these carbs are concentrated in industrially processed food products.

I want to force this point home and need your full attention to explain it to you: whether you opt for the first or the second front, what I'm about to say will play an important role in your dieting, in stabilizing your weight and in safeguarding your health.

If you're not diabetic, your blood contains 1g of glucose per litre. Since your body contains five litres of blood, you have 5 x 1g, i.e. 5g of glucose, which is equivalent to one teaspoonful of table sugar. If you nibble your way through a packet of biscuits, you'll take in over 100g of carbs which will get into your bloodstream within 40 minutes, which then gives you 20g per litre of blood. If your pancreas didn't secrete insulin, this would send you into a diabetic coma and kill you. Yes, this hormone really does save your life because today we eat far too many fast sugars. However, the insulin makes you fat too. When you eat white bread, corn flakes, mashed potato, well-cooked pasta or honey, when you drink sugary fizzy drinks and when you ingest anything containing these violent carbs, the insulin flows freely as it immediately sets about dealing with the alarming rise in carbs in your bloodstream.

The first thing the insulin does is order all the body's cells to burn off the glucose as a matter of priority, by blocking the use of fatty acids in the blood. These fatty acids therefore return to where they get stored, in the adipocytes (fat cells).

The second thing the insulin does is urgently expel the glucose from the bloodstream. And there are only three possible places that will take glucose: the liver, muscles and adipose tissue.

Let's look at this in closer detail. The liver can take in glucose by storing it as glycogen but it has only limited capacity, so if a person is physically inactive very often this space has already been taken up by glucose stored from the previous day. The same goes for the muscles, which are the first cells to use glucose provided they are being worked. If a person is physically inactive, unused glucose stagnates in the muscles, which are then unable to accept any more. Having been expelled from the blood by the insulin and transformed into fat, the excess glucose is almost always sent to the adipose tissue where it ends up in a practically unlimited storage space that can gluttonously accommodate over a million calories!

3. **It reduces the amount of fats**, only because of their high calorie content. We need fats but we only need a little. One gram of fat provides nine calories whereas proteins and carbs provide us with only four calories.

4. **It places great, not to say enormous, emphasis on vegetables**, which, both in the original method and in this second front, you may eat not only as much as you want but 'as much as you can'. They're essential, being packed with vitamins, mineral salts and fibre, and yet are fairly low in carbs.

5. **It puts proteins at the core; they are the foundation**. Proteins are the most filling foods we have. The body has to work hard to digest and assimilate them, greatly limiting the energy we can extract from them. Over the past 70 years they've more or less remained the same. An egg from before 1944 and an egg today are identical. The same goes for beef steak, cod fillet, chicken legs, prawns and crab. What's more, studies funded by the European Commission have proved that maintaining a stabilized weight is dependent on eating a high-protein diet.

What do we notice around us? Our dietary landscape, which underwent such rapid expansion during the second half of the twentieth century, consists of foods made from the third food group: carbs. And, of course, among these we find refined sugar and ultra-refined white flour, but even more worryingly glucose and fructose syrups, which are primarily responsible for our worldwide obesity explosion. Nowadays the danger lies in sugary, starchy foods, biscuit products and, by extension, the huge range of snack products whose glycaemic index (or penetration level into the bloodstream) means the pancreas is attacked head-on and massive quantities of insulin have to be secreted. These snack foods end up as glucose, the energy-giving food par excellence. But glucose becomes a surreptitious poison once the body is mired in inactivity and can barely make use of it, and once the now weary pancreas decreases its insulin production, thereby allowing the basic blood sugar level to rise.

The dramatic increase in the number of overweight people in the world since the 1950s is linked to two biological effectors: serotonin and insulin, whose combined effects explain the intensity of this phenomenon.

Serotonin
Serotonin is a neurotransmitter produced in the brain whenever we adopt behaviour patterns that directly or indirectly protect our survival. We're rewarded for doing this by a feeling of pleasure, and our desire to live gets recharged. Whenever we're deficient in serotonin, we're

not aware of it but we vaguely sense a lack of well-being, which subconsciously drives us to behave in a way that produces serotonin. Despite our conscious annoyance at growing fat, this explains how we're attracted to the most rewarding comfort foods, the ones most able to produce serotonin inside our brain.

Insulin

Insulin works very differently. It is a hormone secreted by the pancreas to control our blood sugar level and keep it at a concentration that prevents any danger to the organs irrigated by the blood. Foods rich in violent carbs that invade the bloodstream force the pancreas to continually step up insulin production because, physiologically, man and his pancreas are not prepared for this kind of attack. This makes us put on weight, and for those of us with a fragile pancreas, it causes diabetes.

To sum up, we can see one and the same causal agent influencing the way these two vital biological substances work: violent carbs or fast-acting sugars. These foods (sugar, white flour, corn flakes, cakes, sweets, cookies, biscuits, fizzy drinks, purées and so on) are just as toxic as alcohol or tobacco and like them they depend on the support of powerful lobbies for their continued development and promotion.

What's more, these 'non-human' foods, which as far as taste is concerned seem so delicious to us, create sensations that our brain processes in the same reward circuits used by the hardest drugs. Neuroscientists are aware that fast sugars are addictive substances. We use them to deal with a lack of well-being, with dissatisfaction and misery. This explains why such foods, which have enough appeal to our senses to be comforting, tend to make those people fat who are vulnerable and struggling through hard times.

Finally, for the same amount of calories, these foods happen to be the cheapest available. This explains why obesity affects first and foremost the disadvantaged, who more than other classes have need of cheap but intense pleasure. The whole circle is completed.

So I believe that sugar and violent carbs are the number one cause not only of the obesity epidemic but of the diabetes epidemic too. Since the dramatic and concurrent surge in both conditions, which have always been studied and classified separately, they've shown how they're intimately connected. They originate from the same causal agent. How they develop depends on the state of a person's pancreas.

If genetically you come from a family that doesn't have pancreas problems, excessive consumption of sugar will over time make you overweight, and then obese if you carry on eating it.

However, if genetically you have a vulnerable pancreas because diabetes runs in the family, you'll put on weight while developing diabetes.

After eating too much sugar over the years, obese and diabetic people who reach the age of 50 or so then find that their weary bodies start to decline. Usually this is the point when major complications arise from being over-weight, problems affecting the cardiovascular system, high blood pressure with the risk of strokes, cancer, sleep apnoea, arthritis, kidney failure and dialysis, amputa-tions, blindness and so on.

How Does the First Front Work?

The original method comprises four phases: two for losing weight, drawing on the strength of your motiva-tion to get you rapidly down to your True Weight, and two further phases designed to prevent you from ever putting weight back on.

The Attack phase lasts four days on average (between three and seven days depending on how much you need to lose). It uses 72 high-protein natural foods of which you can eat as much as you want. Lean cuts of beef and veal, all fish and shellfish with no exception, poultry with-out the skin (but no flat-beaked birds such as duck or goose), eggs, low-fat sliced turkey, chicken and ham, fat-free dairy products and plant proteins such as tofu, seitan and tempeh. To this you also add $1\frac{1}{2}$ tablespoons of oat bran each day, along with a daily 20-minute walk.

The results are astounding: weight loss can vary from 3 pounds if you're 10 pounds overweight, to 10 pounds if you have more than 50 to lose. Getting such quick results is hugely encouraging. It's a powerful and lasting way of boosting a patient's motivation to carry on dieting.

The Cruise phase follows on immediately from the Attack phase and introduces all the vegetables, except for starchy foods. It progresses with weight loss at a couple of pounds a week until you reach your target weight.

To this you add 2 tablespoons of oat bran and a 30-minute walk each day. Should there be any stagnation, increase the walk to 60 minutes for four days.

For example, if you're aiming to lose 20 pounds, you'll need four days in the Attack phase to get rid of 4 pounds and eight weeks in the Cruise phase to achieve the overall loss of those 20 pounds within two months.

The Consolidation phase starts the day you attain your True Weight.

This phase aims to prevent you from immediately regaining the weight you've just lost, the famous 'rebound', by allowing access to a range of foods sufficient to stop you losing weight but not enough for you to put the pounds back on.

How long it lasts is proportionate to how much you've lost, i.e. five days for every pound lost. For example: if you've lost 20 pounds, you'll need to spend 100 days in Consolidation.

The Consolidation phase is divided into two equal parts. If it's 100 days, this means two lots of 50 days.

The first part of Consolidation combines the following foods:

- Proteins are still allowed, as much as you want, as much as you need.

- Vegetables too are as much as you want; not only as much as you need, but as much as you can.

And you add:

- One piece of fruit per day – any fruit except grapes and bananas.
- Two slices of wholegrain or wholemeal bread.
- One 40g (1½oz) portion of cheese, hard if possible, with less than 45% fat.
- One 180g (6oz) portion of starchy foods: al dente pasta (cooked), brown rice, couscous, lentils, cannellini beans and chickpeas. (Avoid potatoes, white rice and overcooked pasta as their fast-invading carbs trigger insulin secretion and make your body store fat.)
- Finally, one celebration meal a week. You're free to choose whatever starter you want, the same goes for your main dish and dessert, and you are allowed a nice glass of wine or a large beer. You can eat what you like at this meal but you mustn't have seconds.

The second part of Consolidation keeps to the same structure as the first; however, it is extended in the following way:

- Two pieces of fruit instead of one.
- Two portions of starchy foods instead of one.
- Two celebration meals a week instead of one.

All foods are here and together they form an ideal model for the human diet. The Consolidation phase is similar to the Cretan diet and the Mediterranean way of eating. And if everyone were able to follow it, it would mean we'd all maintain a normal weight and anyone who had lost weight wouldn't put any back on.

The Stabilization phase is the final phase in my diet. You'll need to be good at managing your independence and the complete freedom to eat once again whatever you like. This phase is the most crucial, because the future of your new weight depends upon it. It's also the most vulnerable since this is when the structure and defined path that kept you on the straight and narrow fade away to make room for three measures, which have been honed down to be as simple as possible so that you can stick to them for the rest of your life.

Basically the only way to win the battle of the pounds is not to put any back on again. Because anyone with weight to lose – and this includes the most extreme cases of obesity – will have at least once in their lives lost their surplus pounds.

If you keep as your reference point the food base from the Consolidation phase, the ideal human diet, it will give you a safety platform to which you can withdraw, should you have any eating lapses that jeopardize your current stability.

During this time, the three measures are simple; they give you the best results for the least possible restriction:

- **Protein Thursdays**, one day a week that's there to protect the other six days. This day allows you to counteract any imbalance. If you're not keeping to your Thursdays, you're slipping up and losing your grip. Managing to keep to them means you're in control.
- **A 20-minute walk every day** and using the stairs instead of taking lifts and escalators. You have to decide to remain active and resist being passive or leading a sedentary lifestyle.
- **3 tablespoons of oat bran a day**. This measure is beneficial, useful and pain free.

These three measures work like a ritual. What's more, they're effective and hardly restrictive at all. Combined, they'll strengthen your motivation so that you don't endanger your True Weight – a vigilance kit, if you like.

I've noticed something that I find very inspiring: anyone who accepts these measures doesn't put weight back on. Often, even very often, they find that their gravitational pull shifts to vegetables and proteins. They're no longer fixated on starchy foods, sweet things and fats. And this happens smoothly, gradually as the days pass following the method, and then quite freely. I've been delighted to see that the range of foods I so carefully spread throughout the different phases remains embedded as something both practical and theoretical. Even when in challenging situations – anything from business lunches to large family gatherings – they're able to negotiate their way around obstacles, avoid excesses and make the protective ritual of Pure Protein Thursdays part of their routine, which guarantees that they'll never regain weight.

Now, you know the essential points of my original method. And in the second front's Nutritional Staircase you'll discover the same principles but applied to the week(s) that you'll need to achieve your True Weight. Afterwards there'll be a Consolidation and Stabilization phase; you'll also find my three pieces of advice for your vigilance and weight control kit.

Pleasure and Serotonin

I now have an exceptionally important gift for you: read the following pages and I assure you that it will change the course of your life.

I'd actually like to pause for a moment here and talk to you about something to which I personally attach the utmost importance. This is a matter that I've thought about long and hard and which has brought me much, not only in my professional work treating weight problems but, even more so, in shaping the way I understand the world and in developing my philosophy of life. I'm very keen to share it all with you, and then you can decide what to do with it.

I'm convinced that it'll help you improve your life, most especially with relation to your weight problems, as being overweight very often suggests some underlying dissatisfaction.

What you are, just as what I am, as far as our bodies, as well as our physiology, physique, mind, emotions, psychology and spiritual aspirations, are concerned, was not programmed for life in the world as we now know it.

Today, when a mother gives birth, she places in its cot a small human being who was designed by the laws of evolution to survive in the environment into which our species was originally born. This child is 'factory programmed' to live in a natural setting that has to be continually overcome otherwise death awaits, a place where nothing can be taken for granted. A world where food is hard to come by and is hard-won. A world with no antibiotics, no machine guns, no concrete, no telephones, no screens, no hospitals, no maternity wards, no social insurance, no cinema and no dating or social networking websites. And, as for what interests us, as far as food goes, a world without any trace of sugar, without any supermarkets – these places with so much food on display that our efforts are channelled in the opposite direction nowadays: we no longer struggle to find food; today we struggle to say no to it.

Yes, this was a time when life was touch and go. No one would wake up safe in the knowledge that they'd still be alive by bedtime; people lived at the mercy of an infected wound, a difficult childbirth, famine or cold. Yet, in this unsafe world you would enjoy the immense pleasure of hunting and gathering in an unspoilt and awesome natural habitat, as well as the solidarity that linked members of the extended family group ensuring that everyone survived. And you would live within this group, bonded to your opposite-sex life partner, who you couldn't be without. And then you'd also be attached to your children and family. All these ties would develop effortlessly alongside the acute, permanent need to survive.

44

This was a group where everyone excelled at doing what he or she did best, with everyone working together, advancing like a frail barque out on to the wide, open sea. A chief who wasn't just the best warrior; the medicine man, a natural healer who knew which gestures and which plants heal; the sorcerer who talked to the gods and to invisible powers; the 'entertainer' who would be merry, sing, dance and mime; and the hunter who understood the language of the animals and only killed them to survive while asking for forgiveness. You'd be desperate to be a part of this group, it's more or less in your blood – being outside it would be totally unsafe and spell certain death.

Your habitat was immense and natural, with space extending as far as the sky and sea. A habitat that protected, a habitat you needed to keep those dear to you safe, a habitat without which you couldn't dream while asleep.

You'd always be aware of your body, you'd use it as your first instrument for survival; your body would feed, protect and defend you. A weapon and a tool you'd enjoy possessing and using, your body is rooted in the sacred. You need your body.

Nature may be hostile but it was nourishing, a birthplace as much as a last resting place, splendid surroundings populated by predators and prey. You'd be a part of this nature which you share with the animals, plants and the elements.

You'd need to play and laugh since this is what makes us human, to come together so we can relax and learn how to live.

Finally, primitive man had an enormous, overwhelming need for the sacred, which made him great – his organic need to believe in a universe governed by invisible but tangible powers, the magic of which governed his life. This irrational need was as vital to him as the beatings of his heart. He interpreted everything based on what he believed without any demand for proof. It was because of this magical spirit that he put up totem poles, decreed taboos and submitted to the forces of gales, winds and thunderstorms and to the commandments of the gods, who merely by being invoked could dissolve the anguish of death. As far back in time as we care to look, man has lived in a world shot through with the sacred.

And to deal with these forces equally revered and feared, man had a synchronous, dual need, an attraction and a biological, even mental, fascination for the language of Beauty, a need to immerse himself in the beautiful, to acknowledge it and, for some, to create it. Beauty spiritualizes everything it permeates.

This is our man, this is Homo sapiens sapiens; this is you and this is me.

This man emerged some 200,000 years ago, produced by the evolution of the species, with transcendental operating instructions that placed him on the very top rung of life's ladder. He then reproduced for over 190,000 years in a world where only those individuals who were desperate enough to stay alive by following the inner voice of their instincts survived and bred.

Nowadays, just like him, we're programmed to respond to these very same instincts, driven by behaviour patterns to seek out pleasure, pleasure that we get whenever we pursue goals that ensure the survival of the individual and of the species.

I'm hungry, I eat, I enjoy what I eat and I survive.

I love a woman, we find pleasure together, we bring forth life and the species survives.

The guidance and synchronicity for our actions are orchestrated in our brains as a magnificent neuronal symphony.

I call the conductor of this symphony the **pulsar**, a primordial transmitter tucked away in the farthest corner of your primitive brain. Very early on, in the comfort of your mother's womb, it starts sending out signals and it never stops, unless you're beset by depression.

Please note that I'm not talking about some generic, virtual or theoretical man, I'm talking about you.

Thus your pulsar, constantly busy, emits the only thing that makes the difference between a living person and one who is dead (or severely depressed): the vital energy that you experience as your desire to live. This energy, or this urge, activates the ten or so **reward-seeking behaviour patterns** that are there to help you live. Their mission is to persuade you to produce a particular reward known as **pleasure**. How we experience pleasure will vary, depending on what our behaviour patterns focus on.

There's a world of difference between pleasure from eating, sexual pleasure, a walk in the forest or reading a good book. Nonetheless, regardless of what pleasure you reap or which path you take, all roads lead to Rome. They have the same mission; and up until about 20 years ago we had no inkling this was happening. The mission is to get our brains to secrete the amazing chemical transmitter substance **serotonin**, which underpins the cornerstone of the human edifice: our taste for life, our desire to stay alive and our need to be alive, without which everything very quickly comes to a halt.

How does this amazing mission get accomplished?

The pulsar provides the energy, the reward-seeking behaviour patterns track down their target, serotonin is produced, it loops back to the pulsar and recharges it, making sure that it keeps on sending out its signals.

This is how men lived before and how we are alive today.

After 190,000 years of 'natural' life, man discovered that instead of hunting animals he could rear them, and that he could cultivate crops rather than gather them. Another mode of human life came into being, one that was safer and longer.

Mankind was now no longer preoccupied with ensuring its immediate survival. The human brain developed and organized itself so that progress followed, and inventions and discoveries as simple but as decisive as the wheel, the sail, the bow, the yoke and metal were made, which gradually brought great improvements to man's daily life.

And this is what went on until 1944, when science, technology, communication, transport and medicine brought about a revolution as significant as the Neolithic revolution, which spelt the end of primitive life. This revolution marked our entrance into a universe based entirely on the economy, one where Growth became the commander-in-chief. In exchange for comfort and entertainment, individuals submitted to the society in which they lived. And from that point on, as the founding principles of mankind were undermined, the priorities of individuals were overshadowed by those of society.

Whereas the human animal's operating model is based on getting enough serotonin because without it man cannot experience pleasure or the need to live, the operating model for our current societies is based on the need for continuous economic growth.

To maintain this growth, our societies have to produce more goods and wealth each year. And so that what they produce gets absorbed, they require their members to consume what they produce. In this type of society, where the economy is like a religion, you're still integrated in your group and you benefit from its profusion, provided you take on your role as consumer. This could all be perfectly legitimate and possible, except that you're not programmed for this role or this fate. The 'human' in you 'resists'.

This means that society has to indoctrinate you so that you adapt to it. It's when we follow these silent influences that we encounter weight issues – the collateral effect of a brainwashing conducted under the crossfire of two incitements.

You'll be aware of the **first incitement** because it permeates your daily life. It uses advertising, marketing, packaging, lobbying, sound, image, words, seduction, sex, fun, competitions, opinion makers and 'as seen on TV' promotions. Although you don't actually need anything, you find yourself going to Thailand on a package tour, taking calls on a second mobile phone while drinking an internationally branded fizzy drink. Experience proves that in the vast majority of cases, we take on this consumer role often believing it to be a sign of progress and part of history's forward advance.

The **second incitement** is more bound up with dissuasion or avoidance. It's hidden, latent and advances stealthily since it's also cynical, immoral and barely acceptable. Quite simply, you are being subjected to society's negative incitement to break away from what's programmed inside you that will make you happy naturally.

And for the simple reason that natural sources of satisfaction are free. Left to follow your own instincts, you'd spontaneously gravitate towards these simple but dense and profound sources of satisfaction.

So What Happened in 1944?

That year the Bretton Woods Agreement sealed a new monetary and economic pact which established a radical change in the human condition: society's functioning and its needs would take precedence over the individual and their needs. From that moment on, everything was set up to ensure that a new type of society could flourish. A society that can only survive by producing and consuming more each year, where there's nothing to ensure fulfilment for the individual.

Let's stop for a moment and look at this new equation for human life. It's very relevant to you, particularly so if you have a weight problem.

Society, speaking through its manufacturers, offers you a huge range of consumer products including food. To be sure, they give you satisfaction, but superficial, short-lived satisfaction, and you grow accustomed to them so quickly that they become necessary. That's how it is. However, at the same time, this pressure to consume is silently but determinedly competing with the satisfaction your brain receptors are waiting for to be able to secrete serotonin, your 'biological reason for living'.

Having reached this point in the book, I'm beginning to wonder whether I've taken you on a rather long digression, reflecting on matters that may well seem to you scarcely related to your concrete concern to lose weight and find out more about this second front which will help you. However, on reflection, I don't think this is the case because I've often taken the opportunity in my books to raise the level of the debate and I've realized – to my publisher's surprise – that my readers are grateful to me for doing so.

I'll always remember what was for me a significant event. I'd been invited to appear on primetime TV for a well-known channel. A few moments before going on set, an assistant came up to me and said: 'Doctor Dukan, please can I ask you to avoid using long sentences and, most importantly, please, please put your ideas across as if you were talking to five-year-olds.' This sort of attitude fills me to my very core with indignation; I'm appalled by what Dalí called the 'dumbing down of the masses'! And I want to believe that you're not scared off by depth of thought – when it's put across with simplicity.

So I'll carry on and, if you're really not at all interested in what lies behind the reasons that have made you over-weight, you can always just head straight to the section that introduces the second front.

Everything that I've just set out here is directly linked to the role of serotonin. This relatively recent discovery, whose impact we haven't yet quite fully grasped, shows us quite simply which paths we should follow, and which behaviour patterns we should use, to want to live and live happily – they've always been there. An individual who has lost the desire to live won't survive for long, and if all the individuals from a species end up without it, the species is destined to disappear too.

How are we programmed to carry on living? By a simple and brilliant system that evolution has used throughout the animal kingdom: attraction and repulsion.

Serotonin is the key element in a brain system that rewards actions and behaviour that protect life and which at the same time boosts our biological, metabolic and psychological, emotional and affective desire to live. Eating, loving, creating, being physically active, playing, getting close to nature, being in your own home, having beliefs, having contact with beauty and belonging to a group, all these behaviour patterns, directly or indirectly, protect life by distancing it from the risks and dangers that stifle it or threaten it. By adopting them, you'll experience satisfaction. This satisfaction will vary according to the path you take, but it will always head for the same effector, the secretion of serotonin, as this is what recharges your life's pulsar.

Conversely, anything that weakens, undermines or endangers life is endorsed by things becoming uncomfortable for you, then unpleasant, anguishing and distressing until they're intolerable – driving you to give up the things and the behaviour patterns that make you feel this way so that you get back on the path steeped in serotonin.

To state it even more clearly, the more serotonin your brain secretes, the more fulfilling your life will prove to be, the more you'll want to keep on living and the more happiness you'll produce.

Unfortunately, neither you nor any other human being is capable of secreting serotonin of their own free will. We need an intermediary to do it; we use the behaviour patterns naturally hard-wired into us, which once they reach their target, activate our brains to release serotonin.

And if you select these behaviour patterns, clearly it's not because you're searching for serotonin, since you're not even supposed to know it exists let alone how it works. It's because you're seeking out this amazing, magnetic sensation called pleasure.

Pleasure is a sensation 'invented' by evolution to induce you to adopt behaviour patterns that protect the venture of life that fills your being. And, working in symmetry, feeling miserable will, conversely, distance you from what may threaten your venture.

Where does this lead us and how does this relate to the problem of being overweight, and to you being overweight in particular? Quite simply, this is the heart of the problem. If you want to lose weight, and particularly if you want to keep it off for good, here is the concrete, decisive crux of the matter.

What you learn here will guarantee that you succeed. I even believe that learning about how your brain works should help you lead a better life, since it's your brain that determines your happiness.

I do hope I've enlightened you about the yawning gap between the priorities of a mercantile consumer society and those of the individual. Our society can only survive if you consume. However, as an individual, you'll only survive if you feel the biological need to do so. The problem lies in the fact that society draws on all the means at its disposal to pressurize you to agree to swap real satisfaction that's simple, natural and tailored to your 'happiness physiology' for superficial satisfaction that's artificial, short-lived and consequently incapable of producing the serotonin you need to live.

The Ten Pillars of Happiness

During my career working as a doctor specializing in nutrition, I've had the opportunity to meet thousands of patients who'd grown fat by using too much food or the wrong food to fill a gap in their lives or compensate for some underlying dissatisfaction. The vast majority of them had no idea of this process and so they didn't talk to me about it; instead they saw themselves as being overweight because of their hormones or family history, an over-fondness of food or lack of willpower.

Over the years, by asking them questions and, most importantly, by listening to what they described, I would often see obstacles at work in their lives, various reasons for getting annoyed or stressed, difficulties in a relationship, lack of affection, sexual isolation, occasionally a money problem, a thankless or tedious job, insufficient living space or a feeling of being unloved. I would then direct and refine my questioning to confirm these leads and to find others.

Alongside the two main traditional sources of satisfaction and comfort, which are pleasure from food and pleasure from sex, I could see others emerge which, whenever they were absent from my patients' lives, seemed to play an important role in their overeating.

What I found passionately interesting was the direct and almost mechanical relationship between losing access to one of these sources of satisfaction and the need to offset the loss through extra comfort eating. This means that a divorce, children flying the nest or redundancy often result in weight gain.

It was through this fascinating research that I was able to identify a certain number of needs, which when satisfied create pleasure, contentment and the desire to live. **Ten sources of pleasure and fulfilment that today I realize represent the ten natural ways of producing serotonin.** Ten fundamental, universal needs found the world over and apparently at any age, most of them existing for animals too: the '**ten pillars of happiness**'. These needs have a role and a function; they're hard-wired into us to encourage us to satisfy them so that we stand the best chance of survival. If we adopt them, we're encouraged by being rewarded; and should we refuse them, we get punished.

This machinery is in your brain and the way it works is so simple and logical that once you've discovered it, it's far, far simpler to lose weight and even simpler to live a better life.

1. The Need for Sexual and Family Love

Alongside the need to eat, this is probably the most essential human need.

Man or woman, you belong to one sexual half of the human race, connected to the other half by sexuality, a sphere governed both by your genes and hormones and the pervading culture around you. Sexuality is made up of attraction and repulsion, constraints and powers that structure your life, fill it and give it meaning. This is the supreme cycle of sexuality with its playful seduction, the serious business of forming a couple, sexual pleasure and its fruits. Like all mammals, human beings are divided between sex and taking care of their young. Without the fascination and power of this need, our species would have long since disappeared. Which goes to show just how crucially important it is. And how vital are the pleasures of being in love, of sexuality and of enjoying a strong, fertile relationship, not to mention the ineffable joy of raising children and caring for family. Serotonin is awash in all these many different relationships. It's difficult to imagine a couple, surrounded by children and relations, who wouldn't feel blessed by happiness.

2. The Need for Social Achievement

Whether consciously or not, like all social animals we strive to find the best possible place in society. I imagine that like everyone else, you feel the need to see your worth acknowledged by others and by yourself. Some achieve this by being naturally dominant, by adopting behaviour patterns and attitudes similar to what we call 'alpha' beings, who are 'dominant' in animal societies. Others have particular manual, intellectual or artistic talents or skills. They can carve out a rather good position for themselves in society using their aptitudes and expertise. Often, they have the ability to set something up or be creative, which earns them gratitude from their peers. Until the exponential explosion that came with progress and technology, human work, however poorly paid and onerous it may have been, would have involved some element of creating and making, and the person carrying it out could take some pleasure in it. This used to be called the taste for 'a job well done', well started and well finished. Nowadays, those who take any delight in working are few and far between. To increase productivity, work has been divided up so we no longer feel part of the whole process, which robs it of its sense and purpose. What's more, employment is hard to come by in times of recession. Losing a job always causes misery.

Satisfaction derived from social achievement has become terribly impoverished. Working no longer has the same sense or dignity. For many people the work they do amounts to nothing more than 'fodder' jobs, which only serve precisely to fuel . . . consumption! Only a tiny percentage of people do their job because they're passionate about it. Yet, it could be possible to plough something back into this vast area of human activity and regenerate it. Whatever you do, it's vitally important that you find meaning in it, that you find an outlet to be creative and responsible and thereby gain satisfaction from it.

3. The Need for a Home

We each need to have a bit of space we can call our own, where we can feel at home, safe, comfortable and relaxed. A space where we can have everything that belongs to us and all the people we love in one place. This place is the same as a den, a hut or an igloo. Films and documentaries that show how native peoples live highlight the importance they attach to their habitat. This protected place satisfies a vital need for safety. In Africa, there used to be trees for sleeping. Sleep specialists have recently discovered that it's very hard to dream in an environment that isn't sufficiently secure – and dreaming is indispensable for life. The rock shelters of the Magdalenian hunter-gatherers on the cliffs bordering the Dordogne river are a striking example of a carefully chosen dwelling place. Their primitive habitat was positioned high up on the cliffside, facing the sun. It allowed them to observe the herds of animals arrive and their position when they set off to hunt them, while at the same time ensuring them total peace and quiet. The lookouts, positioned at strategic points along the river, would raise the alarm if there was an attack.

Nowadays, this immense natural need, and the satisfaction it can bring, comes up against the mundane obstacle of prohibitive house prices – which just goes to show the extent to which modern life frustrates us and forces us to change! And we shouldn't forget those people in our consumerist mega-cities who are forced to sleep on the streets as they don't even have a roof over their heads.

4. The Need for Nature

This is our instinctive need to be close to and in contact with our environment, and our planet in general. Animals have lived on it for around a billion years, and we can't do without it despite the long, patient and gradual process of losing touch with the natural world that culture has imposed on us. A Sunday walk in the woods is a pale reflection of this need. Some people have remained in touch with the joys the earth can offer, with everything that lives on it, with everything that is produced on it. They love animals but in their own way. As a joke, I often say the world is divided into four types of humans: those who love dogs and only dogs; those who love only cats; those who love dogs just as much as cats; and those who love neither dogs nor cats! And there are people who need fauna but also flora, the sky with its clouds, winds, trade winds, north wind and zephyrs, seas and oceans with their storms, forests, sunsets, rainbows, mist and volcanoes – they're attracted to all this and it gives them great pleasure. Such people are vets, zoologists, farmers, herbalists, animal breeders, hunters, landscape painters, gardeners, volcanologists, sailors, yachtsmen, mountaineers, potholers, explorers, climatologists and ecologists.

5. Fun and the Need to Play

The whole mammal world is taken up with the need to play. Have you ever watched kittens or lion cubs? As they take each other on, they're teaching each other, simulating gestures that would kill if they were ever to show their claws. Like all our needs, playing has meaning and essential value for both the individual and the species. Playing encourages us to learn while making it easy to have contact with others. By playing we avoid getting bored and fed up. Playing gives a free rein to our imagination, to the imaginary. We play, laugh, dance, sing and tell each other stories.

Playing is a natural activity that improves our mood, creates ties and reduces aggressive behaviour. Communicating, interacting, learning while playing, living while playing: how appealing it all is! It's the joy the actor, comedian or circus artist communicates. For anyone who's managed to hang on to their inner child, it's the ability to have fun, do silly things, play pranks, play cards, dice, create cartoon books.

Unfortunately, our natural need to play has been narrowed down to the entertainment offered by screens – television, (often violent) video games, the internet etc. – and to lots of different gadgets that very quickly become outdated. Devoid of relationships with other people, the joy of playing grows stale. And despite being expensive, these new games have to be constantly upgraded. When money and the profit motive are involved, playing distorts into addiction.

6. The Need to Belong to a Group

The biological binding force that empowers and cements the group is an immense need. Do you know how a female panther lives? She hunts and survives on her own. The need to belong to a group simply hasn't been programmed into her brain. Eventually she can't even stand her own cubs, so she'll spend just enough time raising them to ensure they can live independently. Now take a look at monkeys, migratory birds, shoals of fish and packs of wolves. Immediately you grasp how we are so much more like them. Tribes, clans, sports clubs, choirs, local committees, societies, trade unions, political parties – we live in groups, in gangs.

This need is a distinctive feature of social species, and is also bound up with immediate survival. If a chimpanzee is excluded from its group, this spells certain death. It was exactly the same for primitive man. A striking example of this is a custom practised by Aboriginal people from Australia. If one member sins beyond the pale, without taking on board the group's threats and reprimands, he is awoken one morning by the chief, the sorcerer and the medicine man, who all three have dug up the 'bone of death'. Brandishing this bone in front of the transgressor while pronouncing the traditional curse is all it takes: the offender, doomed by their banishment, passes away within a few weeks.

Man is a social animal, but some more than others. In the need to belong, humans find a way to truly fulfil themselves. Humans are passionate about laws, prevailing beliefs, customs, religions; they love fashion and they uphold traditions. Today, the extraordinary density of social networks is our contemporary expression of the hunter-gatherer's old tribal clan.

However, at times this need to belong may veer towards conformity and obedience.

This is one of the few needs that society sanctions and actively encourages, since it plays a key role in voluntary submissiveness – and I'm talking here of the constant incitement and demand to consume.

7. The Need to Use Our Bodies

This is one need I've so often talked to you about, when advising you to walk and use the stairs. It evolved with the move from plant to animal life, from immobility to mobility. Whereas plant life lives from its roots and from capturing sunlight in its leaves, animal life has to move to survive, and it has to do this efficiently and cleverly. This is why physical activity receives the ultimate reward: secretion of serotonin. It has been proven that this neurotransmitter is produced in both animals and humans when they're physically active. If mice, who have exercise wheels in their cage, are subjected to stress, they neutralize it by walking or running on their wheels. Brain tissue samples from autopsies on mice confirm that after their muscles have been properly worked, there's a high level of serotonin. For humans, the effectiveness of regular exercise has been compared to that of the main anti-depressants we use. This has been tested on cohorts of depressed patients and, after six months, the results are practically identical. However, we note one advantage as regards exercise. It produces serotonin by adapting it to our requirements and to how our brains work in a way that's completely integrated. The effect medication produces, on the other hand, is linked solely to the amount taken and when it's taken. Unfortunately, physical activity, which does us so much good, is fast vanishing from our daily lives. With cars, television and domestic appliances, gone are the reasons for moving about. Healthy, normal activities become mechanized, replaced by machines, right down to the tiniest things we do. From the car wheel to the keyboard, from the lawnmower to the food processor, technology has practically done away with all the physical tasks we need to carry out. This would be a cause for delight, except that it denies our bodies the mobility they need to remain in balance. The consumer is slowly but surely persuaded to become inactive – a state that is presented as the pinnacle of happiness. Manufacturers strive to justify the unjustifiable, they extol the pleasure of being immobile and an inactive, sedentary lifestyle. Whereas, in reality, what makes us happy biologically is being active and mobile in our everyday lives. And happiness makes us lose weight.

So, because being physically active is one of the ten ways of obtaining serotonin, I'd like to help you fully grasp all the benefits you'll enjoy from using your body. To achieve this, you have no need whatsoever of branded sports gear, a trendy gym, a treadmill, an exercise bike, or GPS to know where you're running to. Such things are all very nice but not vital. It all keeps the economy going but doesn't have the slightest impact on your serotonin. Just go for a regular **half-hour walk every day** and you'll get a boost of serotonin. And I can assure you that you'll feel less of an urge to seek it from food, you'll have less of a tendency to put on the pounds and you'll find it easier to shift them and keep them off for good.

And if you've followed my theory and understood it properly, you'll see that what holds true for physical activity also holds true for the nine other sources of serotonin.

When you think about it, these needs I've just described to you are common to both man and animals. However, **exclusive to humans are two other means** of getting this sublime nourishment, this melodious music that the serotonin instrument sends out – and they are the eighth and ninth pillars of happiness.

8. The Need for the Sacred

Since ethnologists started exploring our planet, we haven't come across a single population or culture anywhere, however crude it might be, that doesn't feel the need to look up to the heavens and bow down. An absolute need to believe without knowing, a yearning for the sacred, for a deity and rites, a huge spectrum of satisfactions and stimulus to live – which we call the sacred.

Between the last ape and the first man appearing, an extraordinary phenomenon occurred: consciousness appeared, the final conquest in the evolution of life. Unfortunately, as man took possession of his consciousness, he became aware of how his life is finite and that he is condemned to die. A revelation of this kind endangered the future of the human race. Evolution responded in a marvellous way by hard-wiring our need for the sacred to be part of our most fundamental needs.

Confronted by his innate, natural anxiety, man then created myths, magic, a belief in the transcendent, heaven, the unknowable, a higher being that through another dimension can explain what prevails in day-to-day life – this is religion, spirituality, the need to believe without evidence that which may defy common sense. This whole realm defines the need we have for the sacred; without it we're nothing more than a bubble of life unavoidably destined to burst before long. There are some people, whose personality and very fibre are so shot through with the sacred, who need it so desperately that everything else pales into insignificance. When this calling is too much of a priority, it becomes excessive, subordinating all life to a model of absolute exclusivity which we find among mystics. For others, it's a way of life that is oriented towards the inner being, immateriality and spirituality and closely connected with the free release of serotonin.

9. The Need for Beauty

At the same time as the sacred, a rather mysterious and completely new phenomenon emerged in the evolution of our species: a natural, universal attachment to beauty. The need for beauty appeared some 100,000 years before our era. For the first time, humans adorned their dead with ochre designs and buried them surrounded by flowers and artefacts to embellish their final journey.

Since Lascaux and Altamira, man has left behind everywhere sumptuous and spontaneous testimony to his cult of beauty. He started collecting beautiful shapes and then wanted to create them himself, and so art was born. Mother goddess sculptures, tools, jewellery, body paintings, sculpted objects and so on. Painting, singing, making music, dancing – man created beauty and used it to cast a spell over the world. This aspiration towards beauty, initially connected with the sacred, and all artistic practices that spring from it, is a very good source of serotonin. I'm not equating beauty or the sacred with simple physical-chemical properties in the brain. Quite the opposite. These neurochemical traces of 'reward' prove the extent to which such needs are an integral part of us – in a simple, effortless, natural and immaterial way. The need for aesthetic harmony and emotion is another fundamental element of our human nature, and to live a full life we must satisfy it. And, as with all natural pleasures, the sacred and beauty are free. Praying, meditating, admiring a sunset, a white pebble, a cherry tree in bloom all cost nothing. And there's the rub. Nowadays, beauty is making way for the utilitarian, stepping aside as the economic model overtakes it. A liking for beauty is ennobling, while the utilitarian enslaves.

If you wish to live without being cut off from happiness, you absolutely have to grasp that all the things that appeal to you and attract you do not satisfy the same needs. You have to learn to distinguish between the natural needs your brain is seeking and the rewards from other, artificial needs, and understand that the satisfaction they offer is also quite different.

Man's real needs have always been those that fuel the ten pillars of happiness. They bring a deep, almost biological satisfaction, rewards that have been put there since the beginning of time to sustain life in us at its highest level. We can recognize the workings of serotonin here.

The needs that society and the market generate and condition in us bear witness to tremendous inventiveness and immense attractiveness. To be sure, they give us amazing yet superficial satisfaction, perpetually renewed but short-lived and without any real power, and so they're unconnected and unrelated to the release of serotonin.

Learning how to tell the difference between these natural needs and artificial satisfaction should be taught at school, since it's a wonderful key for accessing the only real reason that makes life worth living: to lead a really happy life and to want it 'to last'.

I've just set out for you **nine fundamental needs** that frame, inform and reward our human endeavour. I don't believe that there's a single person who could completely avoid the influence of all of them, but it's obvious that these needs don't speak to us all in quite the same way and, even less, to quite the same degree. From the moment we're born until we grow old, each of us responds to the appeal of these nine needs, according to our personal and family background. You've just found out about them, so try and pinpoint which life forces most appeal to you, and through which you can best achieve your own potential and personal fulfilment. Because, without a shadow of a doubt, they'll be your best source of serotonin and a solid bedrock for your reasons to live. Is it love, your family, the relationship you're in? Work? Home? Spirituality? Creativity, art, beauty? Your need for nature? Playing and fantasy? The need to be part of a group? All of them or some of them? Which one dominates? Think about it, see how you can draw on them and you'll soon realize how much they can bring you.

10. The Need for Food

This tenth pillar lies at the epicentre of the issue we're tackling together here, which is our need to eat, to look for and find food, to take enjoyment from it and live from it. **Food is the most immediate and vital need, taking precedence even over sexuality.** Your neurones are programmed to protect this need and reward it in the best way possible. Consequently, as well as the pleasure derived from eating, it's the need that, once satisfied, enables the brain to secrete the most serotonin – sexual orgasm coming a close second.

It was in trying to understand the reasons why my patients had gained their unwanted pounds that I discovered three interrelated explanations:

1. The first has to do with a specific disposition that develops from childhood onwards and finds comfort and consolation in eating.
2. The second concerns temporary or long-lasting difficulties in getting fulfilment from a large number of spheres that provide satisfaction. People who, for

various reasons, find themselves unable to access these spheres make do with food, eating and oral pleasure.

3. I found the third explanation while looking at the background to the weight problem crisis. If, as confirmed by the facts, this crisis emerged for the first time in mankind's history around 1945–50, it is bound to be tied up with the change in lifestyle that occurred at that time: the development of our mercantile or consumer society which we've spoken about.

I noticed time and again that most of my very overweight patients were people who were prevented by their circumstances and our prevailing culture from gaining access to certain sources of self-fulfilment – I'm thinking in particular of unrewarding work, relationship breakdowns and difficult family situations. Seeing these sources of pleasure dry up, they seek comfort wherever they can find it; and the greater the emptiness, the more compulsive the eating.

Such deep dissatisfaction is far from being innocuous; it can't last for long before the desire to live diminishes and depression sets in.

This is the reason why men and women who hate seeing themselves grow fat still do nothing to stop filling themselves with serotonin-producing comfort foods. And, as it so happens, these foods are also rich and therefore fattening.

The solution doesn't lie in reconstructing the world or society, but in understanding how we function so that we can manage to live more naturally in a world that is becoming ever more artificial.

Cultivate those needs to which you feel closest and most connected. No individual derives their satisfaction from all these needs combined; you just need to fill two or three of them to flourish. What's really bad for your weight is when all you have left is food and the telly as substitutes for fun. Regrettably, this is no longer quite so uncommon in a world where relationships are under such stress, work so frequently unsatisfying, housing so hard to come by, nature so far away, bodies neglected, God overlooked, beauty hived off into museums and the group overshadowed by solitude.

My experience as a medical practitioner has proven to me that anyone who is able to access easily some of these great natural sources of satisfaction, and absorb a sufficient dose of serotonin, will not put on weight. In spite of everything, should such a person gain weight under the pressure of persistent, serious stress, they'll lose it far more readily than others. Of course, there are other reasons for weight gain, such as family history and hormonal problems, but for me lack of serotonin is by far the main culprit.

Sex, Food, Power, Home, Play, Group, Body, Nature, Beauty and the Sacred. That's where you've got to go looking. These are the spheres where you should try and fulfil yourself.

Through examining case histories over the years, and from discoveries in neuroscience, brain imagery and how anti-depressants and neurotransmitters in the brain work, I've been able to gain a greater understanding of the fundamental relationship between satisfaction, fulfilment and the desire and need to live. In their own lives, my patients avoided feeling bad by devising a way of feeling good to compensate. They were reproducing in their emotional lives what is a major physiological function – homeostasis, which automatically controls our vital functions. For example, if you don't have enough air and oxygen, straightaway your heart starts beating more rapidly to compensate.

Without realizing it, my patients were subconsciously reacting to the extinction of a certain number of natural sources of satisfaction by turning to excessive use of a different source of satisfaction, one they could better control – food.

This is what led me to advance this 'ten pillars of happiness' theory, and postulate that being overweight could be seen as a symptom of a 'happiness disease'.

Each year, there are more people unable to find a way of achieving fulfilment in our prevailing social model which excludes them from the ten pillars of happiness, their natural sources of satisfaction and self-fulfilment. The people who come to my consultations, and those I've always helped, no longer produce enough serotonin. So, mechanically, biologically and without being fully conscious of it, they're instinctively forced to adopt habits, actions and behaviour patterns capable of producing it.

Those who put on weight easily, and who quickly put it back on again after dieting, are people marked by a vulnerability acquired in early childhood, when they learnt to relieve uneasiness or anxiety first by sucking their thumb and then by using a food substitute. As adults, whenever they're in trouble, feeling stressed or miserable, they revert to pathways and habits that are hard-wired deep inside their primitive brain to produce this liberating serotonin. And their search takes them to those foodstuffs that produce the most serotonin: the most tasty and enjoyable foods.

Sugar, flour, incitement and addiction, consumption, estrangement from our real reasons for living, the very low cost of fattening foods (carbs and fats) and the increasingly high cost of proteins and vegetables – all these reasons combined are making an ever-growing proportion of the population in wealthy nations, and those nations that are growing rich, overweight, obese and diabetic.

If I've gone to great lengths to stress the multiplicity of sources of happiness and if I've explained to you so insistently the role and function of serotonin as we search for our zest for life, it's so that you can draw a practical lesson from it which will be useful for the future of your weight.

In any foodstuff, the nutritional – calories and nutrients – co-exists with the sensory – taste and flavour. If you've put on weight, it's because you've homed in on those foods with the most flavour, texture, creaminess, sugar and fat. And you've done this without even being aware of it, driven by what I call your pilot, which controls in you your ability to keep yourself alive. And if your pilot has done this, it's because some threat was hanging over you, in the same way that if you were gagged, you'd do everything in your power to breathe. You should grow used to the idea that looking after this flame of life is such an important thing for an individual that the conscious person can't be entrusted to dispose of it as they wish. Your pilot is therefore programmed to ensure that your reward-seeking behaviour patterns find their target: pleasure and serotonin.

Living in an environment that values consumption over natural satisfaction, if you go along with this conditioning your pilot will force you to seek satisfaction from whichever natural source is left, to overindulge in food and fun.

Armed with this recent knowledge given to us by neuroscientists, you in turn can influence the pilot's decisions. The answer is simple: take a look at how you live. There's a strong likelihood that, as with most people who grow fat while hating what's happening to them, in your search for serotonin you've come to rely a little too much on food and screen entertainment. Now you are aware that there are ten sources of fulfilment and that the system works on the principle of symbiosis, i.e. when certain sources dry up, the ones that remain have to compensate for them. This is how you've put on weight.

If you want to reverse the process, you'll have to reactivate the other sources you've been neglecting and consolidate other pillars of happiness.

I'm convinced that you are indeed able to revitalize certain areas that until now you left alone simply because you were busy, tired or unaware of what they could do.

Lastly, take some time to answer this one crucial question: what's the most important thing in your life?

You'll then see that everything I've just described is actually far from being a digression. Before committing yourself to a dieting method, it's absolutely fundamental that you understand why you've reached the point of needing to lose weight. To make sure that you fully achieve your target – i.e. losing those pounds that are a barrier between you and your self-fulfilment – it's essential to control the mechanism that generated them. So, if the second front that makes up the Nutritional Staircase is a battle plan, these few pages about serotonin and the ten pillars of happiness will enable you to understand why and how you must carry out this plan. What I most dearly want is to help you regain control of your own body so that you're the pilot once again.

The Two Profiles

We've now reached our goal: opening up a second front to fight weight problems. As the term suggests, it works alongside the first front to reach a wider audience, by appealing to new users to whom it may be better suited than the original method.

For a long time I thought that my initial method was enough, but I overlooked two things. The first is that I devised it with patients who were sufficiently motivated to come to my consultations. The second is that the results I achieved with it were, for the most part, down to a one-to-one relationship that involved me being there to offer empathy and my personal support. When I wrote down my message and method in a book, I did my utmost to preserve this empathy, even reproducing the tone and words I used in my consultations. The book and method became a mass tool and, in return, they gave me a considerable number of very good results that broke with those obtained from previous diets centred solely on calorie-counting. Nevertheless, despite this inspiring breakthrough, I could see its limitations. Some people who read my method didn't embark on the programme; others gave up before reaching their goal.

When you've dedicated your life to an endeavour as important as making your contribution to the fight against a global scourge, you're constantly preoccupied with honing your weapons to achieve ever better results. Since I could only see a dozen or so patients a day, and realizing the extent to which supervision and monitoring can help people who are trying to lose weight, I set up a coaching website. I wrote each one of its 12,000 pages of motivational tips, eating advice and exercise instructions which provided daily personalized guidance. However, what I wanted first and foremost was for this coaching to be interactive, so that the user who received their instructions every morning could report back each evening with their results and say how they'd got on.

With this monitoring, I saw the results improve still further. But only for users who were already devotees of my original method's model and philosophy.

So I gradually became aware of another category of potential users, one I hadn't noticed before for the simple reason that they didn't use my diet, fearing it would require too much effort and commitment.

Some of my patients had regularly asked me to moderate the diet; others would write to me. I read the comments posted on forums and, as I went about my daily life, I'd come across people who found that, for them, my method was too warrior-like, too impassioned and militant; people who were definitely aware of being overweight but who, for various reasons (motivation, personality, character and lifestyle), didn't feel prepared to lose weight with the same passion and commitment as those who succeeded so well with the first front. What for some was the strength of my method was actually putting others off, those who were less interested, less miserable and in less of a hurry to get results.

This is how I ended up distinguishing two different profiles among the overweight, and realizing how up until then I'd only been reaching out to the first profile, the very committed type I met in my personal consultations, people with whom I shared the same all-or-nothing temperament.

I'm going to try and outline these two profiles:

The first profile is someone who is very definitely overweight, commonly needing to lose over 2¼ stone (15 kilos) and suffering physically and psychologically because of it. Very often, this situation develops because of problems at home or at work or some other turmoil. In the background is a childhood vulnerability or hypersensitivity that developed into a 'flight to food' when times get tough. Food that seemingly offers comfort is used to cope with the stresses and strains of everyday life. Despite the ordeal of hating being fat, this explains why the need to eat and neutralize the negative situation is too overwhelming to be given up, let alone be switched over to its exact opposite, a weight-loss diet.

Until the day people from this first profile come to me for a consultation:

'Doctor, I've spent the past three years trying to hide my weight problem, appalled to see these unwelcome pounds keep piling on but incapable of doing anything to sort it. I felt ashamed as I watched the months and years go by without doing anything. I avoided looking at myself without clothes on, I looked away from myself in mirrors and I covered myself up with loose-fitting clothes. My wife/husband, my family and friends all said nothing and I felt paralysed as the days went by.'

And then sometimes all it takes is one incident, one look, a smile, an encounter, a trip, a health check, a comment or a holiday photo and that's the turning point, everything changes dramatically, a sudden decision is made, a rush of strength, vigour and energy surges up from deep within, bringing with it an overpowering need to lose weight. Everything that once seemed out of reach is now simple, obvious, desirable and desired.

I would then hear: 'Recently I've felt a radical change take place inside me. A doorway has opened and I know that I can lose weight and draw on this strength that I didn't have before. I don't know what's happened, but I want to use this strength to free myself from my prison of fat.'

Most of these patients have already gone through this experience, they know instinctively that the favourable wind that's puffing out their sails, this thrilling, unusual energy and control, is not destined to last long. And realizing this, they need a tool, a springboard to make the most of it for as long as possible.

They tell me: 'Doctor, I'm impatient to get going, I want to grab the opportunity to make headway while the going is good and I feel this strength inside me. It's like I'm sitting on a bulldozer that will crush any obstacle in my path. So I'm prepared to do whatever it takes. But please, I beg you, I don't want herbal tea or anything wishy-washy. I want a proper diet, one that works as quickly as possible, with immediate results. I want to see with my own eyes that I can do this and keep my motivation going. Do you get me, Doctor?'

In the vast majority of cases, this sort of patient loses weight without any difficulty following the initial method created for them. They rejoice at succeeding and redis-covering their well-being.

The second profile is quite different.

More often than not here is a man or woman who feels the need to lose weight, but without suffering the distress, misery and impatience that being overweight can cause. Here is a calmer person, less tormented by their extra pounds, and therefore better able to live with them.

What differentiates this approach and sets it apart from the first profile?

Firstly, the amount of weight to be lost. The second profile often lies under the symbolic mark of 2¼ stone; being overweight by between ½ stone and 2¼ stone is easier to carry and less visible.

How people experience being overweight varies widely from one person to the next. Some, often men, do their best to put up with an extra 3 stone and seem able to live with it without feeling too miserable. Whereas for others, being an extra stone or so overweight is sheer torture. What's more, I often get the impression that what I hear my patients say bears no relation to what I actually see on the scales. I can recall instances of very attractive looking women who would talk to me from the other side of my desk as if they'd turned into 'monsters'. I remember one of them saying: 'Since I had my last child I've become horrible, all fat and flabby. I've just got to get rid of it, I can't stand it any longer.'

And a few moments later, undressed and on the scales, I saw before me a woman whose body had a slight covering, but who barely needed to diet for more than a few weeks. It's obvious that this sort of patient is at the end of her tether and so miserable that she belongs to the first profile, regardless of how many pounds she needs to lose. Yet, you mustn't go thinking that the second profile isn't affected by being overweight; it's just that they tolerate it with a little more patience and a little less misery.

However, and I see this quite often, second-profile patients classified as able to put up with their weight may move over into the first profile if their weight increases over time and passes a certain threshold, in particular when it goes over 2 and then 3 stone.

Furthermore, second-profile people are usually less vulnerable than first-profile people, their feelings and emotions are not quite so intense; and their weight doesn't impact on their mood and daily lives to the same extent.

How the weight is distributed is another important point. If it's evenly distributed, it's easier to tolerate. However, what is hard to live with, sometimes to the point of obsession, is a big stomach for men, and big rounded hips and thighs for women. Terms such as 'cellulite' or 'paunch' reflect how much this localized accumulation of fat is loathed. Cases like this are almost always found in the first profile, whereas with the second, weight is more evenly distributed.

So this is how a second-profile female patient using the second front describes herself:

'Doctor, I know I need to lose some weight – nothing new there because I've been battling with these pounds for ages – but to tell you the truth I've never really gone for it. It's never really got me down so much that I've wanted to throw myself into a very strict diet. I'm not in any particular hurry.'

Another example: 'I have to confess that I like the good things in life and my husband has never remarked about me being overweight. I also lead a really busy social life, I've got a big family and I'm out all the time, especially at weekends. That's how my life is and, to be frank, I just can't see myself making dramatic changes and giving it all up.'

And another: 'I think I'm healthy and don't feel in any danger. I don't have diabetes or high cholesterol, so no real reason to follow too strict a diet.'

And even: 'I'd really like to slim down and I'm too sensible to think I could lose weight without dieting, but

I don't think I'd be capable of following a diet if I wasn't allowed a little treat from time to time. I'd find it extremely hard, for example, to cut out bread altogether and always have to say no to a glass of wine.'

For a long time, I went for the all-or-nothing approach, believing that the diet I'd created suited anyone who had a real need and real reasons for losing weight. And whenever I came across someone who was less determined, I thought that all that was required to get them to accept the method as I'd devised it, i.e. my first front, was to be a little more insistent and offer more support by getting them to report back more frequently.

However, in among the several patients with a real fighting spirit, proud of their results and always ready to do battle, there would be one who'd run out of steam with my diet and who, after following a stage steadfastly and successfully, would ask for a little respite, hoping for some small, well-deserved reward. This would be expressed in requests such as: 'Can I add a bit of corn-flour to my oat bran galettes or a tablespoonful of fat-reduced cocoa to my home-made custards?'

When I started working as a nutritionist, I was very young; I wanted to innovate, and I needed to establish my authority as supervisor and therefore show how tough I was, although this isn't in my true nature. This meant that I was a stickler back then for what I consid-ered to be 'lapses'. However, with time and age, and most especially the confidence that comes from experience and my method's results, I wanted to give some pleasure to these men and women who were close to exhausting their motivation under the strain.

And so I was all too happy to grant them these small permitted departures, which I believed were one-offs.

All too often, though, the news would get out the next day on a blog or a forum or a website and the permitted departure would then become part and parcel of the method.

This illustrates how I built my method, over time and through constant interaction with my patients, then with my readers and the vast community of internet users.

This is how the list of 'Dukan Tolerated Foods' came about, which I ended up incorporating into the method, to prevent mealtime monotony from eroding my patients' motivation. These ingredients can be used to liven up your daily fare and add a bit of variety. These foods contain a little more sugar or fat than the ones allowed, but as you can only have a maximum of two portions a day, you won't stop losing weight. (Please note that you can only have them from the Cruise phase onwards and they're not allowed on Pure Protein Thursdays.)

Tolerated Foods

- Fat-free plain Actimel (1)
- Fat-reduced, sugar-free cocoa powder, 1% fat (1 teaspoon/7g)
- Crème fraîche max. 4% fat (1 tablespoon/30g)
- Soy flour (1 tablespoon/20g)
- Ready-to-use gazpacho (1 glass/150ml)

- Low-fat coconut milk, less than 15% fat (100ml/3½fl oz)
- Soya milk (2 glasses/300ml)
- Powdered skimmed milk (3 tablespoons)
- Cornflour (1 rounded tablespoon/20g)
- Merguez sausages, well pricked and well cooked (50g/1¾oz)
- Ricoré chicory coffee (1 teaspoon/7g)
- Sweetened soy sauce (1 teaspoon/5g)
- Chicken sausages, max. 10% fat (100g/3½oz)
- Fat-free cordials (20ml/¾fl oz)
- Tempeh (50g/1¾oz)
- Cooking wine, for cooking without a lid (3 tablespoons/30g)
- Fat-free fruit yoghurt (1)
- Plain soy yoghurt (1)

It was with the same idea in mind of adapting my method to suit a less determined public with a less heroic profile that I came up with the famous 'Jokers' on my coaching website.

I've explained how my online coaching is interactive and how the subscriber sends back a report each evening answering seven questions. One of them is: 'What food have you most missed during the day?'

And once the yearned-for food has appeared five days in a row, the subscriber is sent a Joker so that they can get relief from their craving. So if someone has told me for five consecutive days that they're missing pasta, their following day's instructions give them the option of making a supper dish with 200g (7oz) of al dente pasta, a nice tomato sauce, all the vegetables they want and a table-spoon of Parmesan cheese. They can then finish off their meal with two yoghurts and nothing else, no proteins.

Likewise, if there's a craving for fruit, I send a Joker for 800g (1lb 12oz)of fruit and two fruit yoghurts for supper.

By experimenting with and trying out ways of making my method more flexible, I observed two predictable facts. Anyone who deep down really wants to lose weight and do it as effectively as possible deems these measures demotivating. One of my female patients told me quite abruptly one day: 'Doctor, I don't need these Tolerated Foods or Jokers. I want to succeed because what's driving me on is seeing that I can get the better of my enemy. It suits me better if this is hard-won, rather than it being handed to me on a plate.'

For her, losing weight was the reward. A good example of the first profile!

Yet there were others who found that even these soften-ing measures didn't go far enough. They'd tried to follow my diet and kept saying: 'You're asking too much of us.'

For them, losing weight seemed like a punishment. They belonged to the second profile.

I had here two very different groups. For one lot, losing (weight) was about winning; for the second lot, losing (weight) was once more about losing. What for some was fuelling their success and was the reason for it, for others was too difficult.

Another factor was the media, which adores fads and does its best to create them. Having supported the most rigid diets for so long, it pressed the pause button – exemplified by the Weight Watchers advertising slogan 'Stop dieting and start living', which is nothing more than a marketing device. Since the 1960s, what has set this American company apart is its group meetings and support – not its diet, which from the very start to this day has remained the same, based on low calorie counts or a 'points' system. So, despite what the slogan might suggest, it's the meetings that help people accept their restricted-calorie diet.

Finally, add to this equation the diehards upping the ante, for whom all diets should be thrown away, regardless which ones. As far as supporters of this idea are concerned, the only solution for tackling any weight or obesity problem is to revert to the body's natural sensations – that is, you should differentiate between hunger and satiety and only eat when you really feel hungry and stop once your hunger disappears. You might as well tell an alcoholic to drink only when they feel thirsty!

When the climate becomes demoralizing like this, many overweight and obese people with very serious health problems grasp the excuse to put off their decision to diet. But these men and women, suffering from diabetes, high blood pressure, cardiovascular, brain or kidney problems or breathing difficulties, need to know that time is not on their side.

Nevertheless, I'd be lying to you if I said that I remained impervious to this 'down with diets' debate. After a lifetime spent fighting weight problems, I could see the danger and the complications, and, as a doctor, I was worried about the risk of demotivating anyone who was still unaware of the threat hanging over them. It's true that a slogan such as 'Stop dieting' has something enticing about it, especially when it seems to promise the possibility of losing weight without any effort. However, when I looked at the social networking sites, blogs and forums, I was relieved to see that there were still as many people out there just as determined as ever to fight for a healthy weight, a nice figure and a positive self-image.

At the same time, I've also been listening hard to people who say that my diet is too strict, and who've therefore let themslves be coaxed away by the dream merchants and their easy come, easy go message. I've paid careful attention to the criticism and objections. Apart from some biased and unfounded comments, other criticism was sensitive, relevant and genuine. It covered the arguments I set out for you when comparing the two profiles. The remarks came mostly from women who'd tried in vain to follow my diet.

I was glad to hear these grievances and requests, and I thank everyone for them. They're constructive, they're truthful and they're heart-felt. So they've helped me hone and improve my way of fathoming how to fight weight problems, which are such a plague that not to do battle would be tantamount to deserting or collaborating with the enemy.

So I worked away furiously to finish off the work I'd started around 2007 based on what I had called the Nutritional Staircase, a more gradual, more didactic, more enjoyable and more relaxed approach. My aim was to provide an answer for anyone needing to lose weight, who knows they need to lose it, who wants to lose it but lacks the right momentum and motivation when it actually comes to it.

For some, their motivation hasn't yet quite reached its peak; however, waiting for it to do so means putting up with these extra pounds and running the risk of slipping into obesity.

For others, it's about something quite different, an emotional vulnerability that seeks consolation or solace in comfort food, which can't be brought under control too brutally, and especially not over too long a period.

It was based on these observations that I ended up dividing my method in two.

Naturally, I kept the existing one, my original method, 'the strong way', which became my first front, my first line of attack.

And I created the second front, 'the gentle way', for people who needed a less full-on but equally effective approach.

Before describing in detail how to use this second front, here's a summary comparing the two profiles that'll help you work out where you fit in.

Comparing the First- and Second-front Profiles

First-front Profile – the Original or 'The Strong Way'

1. Powerful motivation.
2. In a hurry to lose weight quickly.
3. Determined, an all-or-nothing character who does nothing by halves and wants to lose weight quickly to keep up their motivation.
4. Heavily overweight or obese (by over 2¼ stone/15 kilos).
5. Health risks – cardiovascular, diabetes, cholesterol, knee and hip joint problems.
6. A reasonable social life.
7. Robust constitution, quite high or normal blood pressure.
8. A strong liking for high-protein foods and vegetables.
9. Capable of sticking to a strict diet without faltering; able to give up wine, bread and chocolate for a fixed two- or three-month period.

Second-front Profile – the Nutritional Staircase or 'The Gentle Way'

1. Motivation is moderate or hasn't yet reached its peak.
2. Not in a hurry to lose weight.
3. A measured, balanced character, less given to extremes; wants to lose weight but gradually, at own speed.
4. Moderately overweight, often below 2¼ stone (15 kilos).

5. No apparent health risk or family history of cardiovascular disease or diabetes.
6. Busy social life.
7. A weak constitution prone to fatigue; blood pressure tends to be low or normal.
8. Moderate or slight liking for proteins and vegetables.
9. Difficulty keeping to a strict diet over time. Losing weight is more likely through rewards than through tougher instructions.

II

THE SECOND FRONT

or

'The Gentle Way'

The Nutritional Staircase

This new programme, this second front, has been tried and tested by many people, and the results are outstanding. The programme is founded on the same principles, the same values and the same philosophy as the first front. However, its structure, approach and development are different; and, for those adopting it, the fact that it's new has inspired enthusiasm and ownership.

How is this second front different from the first?

As I've told you, the first front, the original method, 'the strong way', is made up of four phases, two for losing weight and two for keeping it off for good. During the first two phases, the prescription is simple: you're allowed as much as you want of 100 foods, 72 proteins and 28 vegetables, until you attain your True Weight. These two phases last several days or weeks. Then you move into the third phase, Consolidation; and you finish in permanent Stabilization, with a complete and varied diet, as well as three precautionary measures for the rest of your life.

THE WAY YOU FOLLOW THE SECOND
FRONT IS TOTALLY DIFFERENT.

It's based on a time unit of one week. One week, from Monday to Sunday. I imagined it as a staircase with seven steps, one for each day of the week.

With each day, the décor changes. With each new step, a food group appears and is added to the previous one. So, step by step, moving upwards, the way opens out to include increasingly rewarding foods. Food groups are added in sequence, starting off with what's most vital and most nutritious – like an open fan, ranging from the most slimming to the most rewarding and liberal foodstuffs. The week finishes off with a flourish, with its celebration meal, and then everything starts again on the next day, on Monday. You'd be hard put to find a livelier and less monotonous diet.

This staircase structure for the second front is designed to be didactic: the idea is that you learn while losing weight. Step by step, and week by week, it goes over the same ground, thereby showing you in a very concrete way the strategic importance of foods as well as the choices to make in order to stabilize effectively. Once you've attained your True Weight, this repetition will have instilled in you a number of useful habits and automatic reflexes. Reinforced week after week, these good habits will allow you to incorporate into your routine a certain amount of theoretical information about nutrition.

I told you about how I used to get enraged with people who would refuse to even accept the idea of dieting. They claim we have a natural system inside us controlling hunger and satiety, and that to slim down to a healthy weight all we need to do is follow its signals.

This system did indeed exist and, with its signals and its sensations, it played a significant role at a time when man was ruled by necessity, tortured by hunger and had to spend every minute of every day thinking about how to glean a few calories to survive. However, today we couldn't be further removed from this scenario; we find it hard to protect ourselves from the abundance around us. Moreover, people who eat too much and so often that they get fat aren't trying to feed themselves. They're using food as an antidote to a malaise and to an existence that, even if it seems acceptable, isn't giving them what their deepest nature is calling out for.

Nowadays, hunger and satiety can no longer play their original role with overweight people. These sensations are operating like locks that have been 'forced'. Few of us eat because we're driven by hunger; on the contrary, we mostly carry on eating without feeling any at all. What's more, not only is food easily accessible now, but it's produced to be enticing, tempting and mesmerizing. Some food has been 'invented' to be addictive, so that its users get hooked.

The Emergency Stairs or Check the Carbs

Take a traditional biscuit and read the label – what do you see? White flour and sugar, and, depending on the brand, a little or a lot of fat. The elements that appeal to our senses – taste, chemical composition, pure sugar and glucose content, consistency and texture, intense flavours – are manipulated in the interests of behavioural marketing. Specialists are at work here, turning these products into proper soft drugs when consumed in small amounts, and harder drugs when eaten repeatedly in larger quantities.

Some psychologists opposed to diets denounce what in their jargon they call 'cognitive restraint'.

What does this term mean? Restraining ourselves cognitively just means understanding that our physiology and primitive reflexes are not enough to protect us. So to help ourselves, we need to turn to our cognitive powers. When our sight fails, we don't think twice about wearing glasses; when our memory starts to fade, we fill up notebooks and computers. So why refuse to read the labels on food to find out what it contains and draw on our knowledge of healthy eating to find our way around this Aladdin's cave that our supermarkets have become? It won't disable us and even less will cognitive restraint make us obese. What's the point of this discussion and who is it aimed at? At the people selling us sugar, chocolate, snack products, fizzy drinks, sweets and creamy puddings.

If you're reading my book, it's because you have a weight, image and possibly a health problem. I beg you to listen to me: be suspicious of sugar. If you take away just one message from what I say, let it be this: **sugar is dangerous for you, for your children, for your family**. If you love sugar, treat it like drinking or smoking. Be aware that one day you'll have to view it as a high-risk food and therefore you'll have to cut down your intake.

The foods I'm talking to you about, these violent sugars and carbs used to make the enormous range of processed snack products currently available, didn't exist 200,000 years ago when mankind came into being, or 8,000 years ago at the start of the Neolithic period, or even when Jesus was alive. They still didn't exist 2,000 or even 1,000 years ago, or when Henry VIII was on the throne. White sugar, extracted from sugar beet, has only been processed on an industrial scale since the mid-nineteenth century. Primitive people from the Amazon or Australia used to eat 2–3 kilos a year. Nowadays, the average American consumes 72 kilos a year, and we see the damage.

With this in mind, I've started a movement called 'Check the Carbs'. I'll explain it to you in the hope that, if I win you over, you'll follow my lead. Take an everyday example. You're about to buy a packet of biscuits for yourself or your children. It's at this point that I'm asking you to Check the Carbs. There's a statutory obligation for any industrially manufactured food product to display its nutritional values on the packaging. Usually there's a box that looks like this:

Per 100g
Energy in kcal
(forget the kjoules, they don't concern you)
Protein
Carbohydrate of which sugars
Fat of which saturates
Fibre
Salt

Find the line 'Carbohydrate': the carbs content is given per 100g of product. I've listed all the snack products sold in supermarkets to compare their violent sugar content (flour and sugar). You may well think that most biscuits contain more or less the same amount of carbs. Well, no, in France it can be double, i.e from 40g to 80g, rarely less and rarely more.

At 80g, you find biscuits, cereal bars, corn flakes. Cynically they're often presented as 'high energy' foods, or are even sold with a 'health food' label. For diabetics, they are real poison; and for the overweight or obese, they're the main reason for their fat reserves.

At 40g, there's still 60g that isn't carbs and such products are very high in the protective fibre that stops the carbs getting into the bloodstream too quickly. For these products to have such a low level of carbs, they can't be made with refined sugar. Instead, traditional sweeteners such as maltitol have been used. They do contain a few carbs, but they're extremely slow ones and hardly impact on your blood sugar level. So for diabetics and anyone watching their weight, these products are particularly recommended. You can recognize them from the statutory wording 'sugar free' or 'no added sugar', the same as with chewing gum and diet fizzy drinks.

My aim is for you to be informed, so that you can decipher these figures, which are far from being a mere detail. One life is 90,000 meals. Repeating the same mistake with your food over the years can have a major impact on your health. Especially so, given that a product may well have been manufactured following rigorous procedures, in totally hygienic conditions, using impeccable products and with complete traceability. However, if you eat too much of it, this product may turn out to be dangerous for your health. Some manufacturers pride themselves on their nutritional expertise, but sell so-called 'health food' products with violent carbs at levels that can easily reach 70g per 100g! This is far too high! Don't let yourself be taken in. You're free to make your own choice, as long as it's an informed choice. This is why I'm campaigning for you to 'Check the Carbs'.

The second line has the words: 'of which sugars'.

This 'of which sugars' is the amount of refined sugar, sucrose, which has been added in 100g of the product. Nowadays, this added sugar in our food is a real danger. I'm not saying that we shouldn't ever have any, but, as with fast driving, you run a risk. And if this risk is taken every day and several times a day, in large amounts, the potential for putting on weight becomes immense. And if a member of your family (uncle, aunt, parent) is diabetic, the chances of you too becoming diabetic are significantly higher.

So my advice to you is 'Check the Carbs'. I do for my children, my friends and most especially for my patients. Whenever I meet a reader, patient or website user who has lost weight with my method and has managed to keep it off, I always ask them what in their opinion has most helped them to avoid regaining weight. They almost all answer that they try to keep away from sugar: 'I eat less than before and I eat more protein foods and vegetables.'

Monday

If you want to follow this second front, you have to start it on a Monday. No matter which day of the week you decide to give it a go, wait until a Monday to get started.

Monday is the first step on the Nutritional Staircase, which has been devised to make up one whole week.

On Monday, D-Day, you'll be allowed to eat all the foods I'm going to list in the following pages, which are all about this first day of the first week.

These are high-protein foods and I've sorted them into **12 categories**.

During this first Monday, you may eat all the foods on this list. You can eat as much of them as you want and when you want – there's absolutely no restriction on quantities or time of day.

You're also free to combine these foods however you wish. So this means you can pick the ones you like and leave out the ones you don't care for. You can even eat just a single food category throughout a meal or even the day.

However, what is essential is that you don't stray from this list as it has been worked out to the very last detail.

As you'll see, you have a really wide choice. However, for this first day, the most important one of all the days we're going to spend together, **you must not succumb to a single lapse.** Were you to stray over the line, even if by only the tiniest margin, it would be like pricking a balloon with a needle. Any lapse, no matter how harmless it seems, would be enough for you to have to renounce your freedom to eat as much as you want, which is invaluable. For just a tiny bit of quality, you'd be losing what you gain in quantity. And for the rest of that day, you'd have to start meticulously counting your calories and restricting your intake – which is the very opposite of what I expect of you.

So, to sum up, the instruction is simple and non-negotiable: you can eat anything mentioned on the list below as it's all yours, but anything that does not appear on this list is off-limits, so for the moment just forget about it. Remember that from tomorrow, Tuesday, I'll be adding another food group to your list.

The 12 Food Categories for MONDAY

1. Lean Meat

I have three types of lean meat in mind: veal, beef and rabbit.

- Beef: you're allowed any cuts you can grill or roast, in particular steak, fillet, sirloin, roast beef and good quality lean cuts. Take care to avoid rib-eye steak and rib of beef as both are too marbled and fatty.
- Veal: veal escalope and roast veal are recommended, and calf's liver too if your cholesterol level can cope with it. You may also eat veal chop, as long as you remove the fat around it.
- Rabbit: a lean meat that can be eaten roasted or cooked with mustard and low-fat fromage frais.
- Pork and lamb *are not permitted.*

You can prepare these meats in whatever way you prefer, but you mustn't use any fat, which means no butter, no oil and no cream, even if it's low-fat.

To preserve the grilled meat flavour, sprinkle a few drops of oil on to your frying pan and then wipe away with kitchen paper.

I'd recommend that you grill your meat, but other options are to roast it in the oven or on a roasting spit, bake it wrapped in foil or even boil it.

It's up to you how long you cook your meat; remember, though, that as it cooks, it gradually loses its fat content.

Raw minced meat is permitted. But make sure that no oil has been used to prepare meat served as tartare or carpaccio.

If you tire easily of eating chunks of meat, then minced meat or burgers are a good bet. Mix together some minced meat with an egg, herbs and capers, then shape the mixture into balls, cook them in the oven and you have a tasty alternative to plain meat.

Frozen steaks are permitted, but do make sure that the fat content is no greater than 10% as 15% is really too high.

Remember, too, that kosher minced beef is full of fat so it's far better to buy some lean steak and mince it yourself. Otherwise, if you cook the meat well enough, it will release some of its fat.

At the risk of repeating myself, let me point out again that there's no restriction on quantities with these foods.

2. Offal

Only the tongue, kidneys and liver are permitted: beef, calf and chicken liver.

You can eat calf's and lamb's tongue since they're lean. As for ox tongue, only eat the front part and especially the tip as it's the leanest bit, but avoid the back part as it's too fatty.

Liver is packed with vitamins, but with cholesterol too, so be sensible if you're sensitive to dietary cholesterol.

3. Fish

There's no limit or restriction as far as this food group is concerned. You can eat any fish you like, whether it's oily or white, fresh, frozen or tinned in brine (but not in oil), smoked or dried.

- All oily fish are permitted, in particular sardines, mackerel, tuna and salmon.
- All white fish are allowed too, such as sole, hake, cod, sea bream, red mullet, skate, trout, sea bass, whiting, plaice, monkfish and many other lesser-known fish.
- You may also eat smoked fish, especially smoked salmon, which although rich and glistening, contains hardly any more fat than a 10% fat steak. The same goes for smoked trout, eel or haddock.
- Tinned fish is very handy for a quick meal or a snack and is allowed so long as it's in water or brine for tuna or salmon, in white wine sauce for mackerel or in tomato sauce for sardines.
- Finally, seafood sticks (surimi). Japanese in origin, they are made from extremely lean white fish and flavoured with crab sauce. Many of my patients and readers are prejudiced against seafood sticks because they are a reconstituted food. But, having looked into how they are made, I know that they also have a high nutritional quality. The tiny white fish are processed on factory ships immediately after they've been caught.

Others have pointed out to me that the labelling

indicates that they contain a small amount of carbs. This is true; however, it doesn't rule them out since we're talking about starch here and the other ingredients are so beneficial that I can tolerate this. In fact, seafood sticks are very low-fat and are extremely handy as they're easy to carry with you, odour-free and don't require any preparation or cooking. You can snack on them at any time of the day.

You must prepare your fish without adding any fat (use 3 drops of oil wiped away with kitchen paper). So either sprinkle over some lemon juice and seasoning or stuff your fish with herbs and lemon or cook it in a court-bouillon – but if you can, try and steam your fish. The best option still is to cook your fish wrapped in a foil parcel as that way you get all the cooking juices.

4. Seafood

In this food category, I group together all crustaceans and shellfish.

- Prawns and shrimps, Mediterranean prawns, gambas, crab, lobster, crayfish, Dublin Bay prawns, cockles and whelks.
- Oysters, mussels, clams and scallops.

You should remember to keep including these foods as they add variety and a touch of festivity to your diet. Seafood also makes you feel nice and full.

5. Poultry

- You can eat any poultry except flat-beaked birds (duck and goose) – but only if you never ever eat the skin. However, you have to cook the bird with its skin on so that the meat doesn't dry out; but once it's on your plate you must remove all the skin.
- Chicken is the most common and practical poultry available. You can eat any part except the outer part of the wings, as this is inseparable from the skin and too fatty. There is a marked difference in the fat content of the different parts of a chicken and the breast is the leanest meat, followed by the drumstick and then the wing. Lastly, your chicken should be as young as possible.
- Turkey in all its guises, pan-fried escalopes, or a drumstick roasted in the oven studded with garlic cloves, or a turkey crown.
- Guinea fowl, pigeon and quail are permitted, as are waterfowl and game birds such as pheasant, partridge and even wild duck, which is a lean meat.

6. Low-fat Cooked Meats, Without Rind or Fat

Nowadays, you can find low-fat cooked ham, chicken and turkey in most shops and supermarkets. They have a fat content between 2% and 4%, which is far lower than the leanest fish and meat. This means that low-fat cooked meats are permitted and I really do recommend them since they are so readily available and easy to use.

The same applies to bresaola or air-dried/wind-dried beef, which is lean and tasty but can also be expensive.

You'll find vacuum-packed cooked meats in any supermarket, but they taste far better and less salty if you go to your butcher or delicatessen and ask for a few slices.

Packaged, pre-sliced, odour-free and waste-free, you can easily take these meats with you and use them to create your lunch. What's more, even if they don't quite rival delicatessen meats in flavour, their nutritional value is comparable in every respect. However, I should remind you that other deli hams and cooked meats are not allowed, in particular smoked or cured hams, which are much fattier.

7. Eggs

Eggs can be eaten hard-boiled, soft-boiled, fried, as an omelette or scrambled in a non-stick frying pan, i.e. without adding any oil or butter (use 3 drops of oil and wipe with kitchen paper).

To ring the changes and provide a little sophistication, you can add a few prawns or even flake in some crabmeat. You could also make a Spanish-style tortilla, using some chopped onions or a few asparagus tips by way of flavouring.

Since the foods I'm allowing you to have are at your discretion, eggs may pose two problems related to their cholesterol content and tolerance. Eggs are high in cholesterol, so if you're sensitive to this you should be careful how many you eat. You ought not to eat more than four yolks a week. However, since egg whites are one of the healthiest foods we have, you can eat as many as you like.

If you're preparing scrambled eggs or omelette, try to use one yolk for two whites.

Some people do have a genuine allergy to egg yolk, but this is extremely rare and generally they have been a sufferer since childhood and therefore know how to avoid it. What is far more common is that eggs are badly digested, which we mistakenly think is due to a fragile liver. If we discount eggs that are too old or off, it isn't the egg itself that the liver can't take, but the cooked butter in which the egg is prepared. So if you're not actually allergic, and if you cook without any fat, you may eat one or two eggs on Mondays without any risk.

8. Vegetable Proteins

Over recent years, an increasing number of vegetarian patients have asked me to adapt my method to fit their requirements. This is why I've introduced and gradually expanded this high-protein but vegetable-based food category. Most of these soy- or wheat-based vegetable proteins come from the Far East, and in particular from Japan. They've become popular here in the West as we're so keen on Japanese food and restaurants at the moment.

In this eighth category I've included seven very low-fat but high-protein foods. However, only the first two, **tofu** and **seitan**, made from soy and wheat respectively, contain enough protein for you to eat 'as much as you want' of them, just as you can with the previous seven categories. Although the five other foods, tempeh, vegetable burgers, textured soy protein, soy milk and yoghurt are very useful, I'm reserving them for vegetarians who eat neither fish nor meat.

Tofu

Making your own tofu is quite easy and enjoyable: grind soy beans in some water to produce soy milk and then add salt to make it coagulate and produce firm tofu with a cottage cheese-like texture. To make silken tofu, you just have to add a coagulant called 'nigari' and heat up the mixture. If you fancy having a go, you'll find lots of cookery websites with information about both types of tofu.

For those of you who don't want to keep repeating this procedure time and again, tofu is now readily available in supermarkets, organic food stores and Asian shops.

Silken tofu: a cooking ingredient with the consistency of custard or yogurt. Sold in packets at room temperature, it is best kept in the fridge for up to three or four days. It's particularly useful in cake and dessert recipes, or for quiches with an oat bran base, and it's great in sauces where it acts as a substitute for mayonnaise or cream. Given its consistency, it can be whipped up to rival any Chantilly cream.

Firm tofu: this has the consistency of firm cottage cheese and can be used in a whole range of recipes. You can eat it crumbled, grated, cubed or puréed in any sort of main dish, starter or pudding. It has little flavour itself, but it soaks up all the flavours of the other ingredients it's cooked with. It goes really well with chives, soy sauce and mild spices. Add tofu cubes to your mixed salads, or to vegetable tarts made with oat bran. Before you start cooking with it, it really pays to marinate the tofu for a few hours in the sauce of your choice. So that it absorbs all the flavours from the marinade, first get rid of any water: you can do this by pressing it between two plates, with the top one weighted down.

Like mozzarella, firm tofu is kept in the fridge and in some water which should be changed every couple of days. Don't keep it for longer than ten days. Tofu is gradually becoming commonplace in the West, a little like surimi seafood sticks, and has an important place in my method. You can now find tofu with herbs or smoked, as well as a range of tofu recipes, from Provençal tofu to curry and poppy seed tofu and saffron tofu. You can also find tofu-based meals, tofu ravioli and tofu sausages. However, remember that these products and meals have not all been cooked following our dietary principles, so you should check the labels very carefully and avoid anything with a fat content greater than 8%.

Seitan

Seitan, or 'vegetable meat', is the equivalent of tofu but made from wheat instead of soy proteins. Its crunchy texture is not unlike meat and it can be used in most stews and casseroles, as well as for kebabs and fricassées. You can buy it ready to use, plain or flavoured, from organic and Asian food stores.

It's also cheap and simple to make seitan at home; if you have the time and inclination, it's fun and empowering to produce your own. You wash wheat flour in a fabric bag to remove all the starch, so that you're left with only the gluten. If you don't have time, buy it ready-made, but don't skimp on preparing it properly. Seitan started off as an organic food aimed at vegetarians. However, I think it's time it reached a much wider public, and especially anyone on a diet who wants to broaden their choice of foodstuffs.

Nutritionally, seitan is extremely high in proteins (25%), low in fat (110 calories per 100g); it contains only very few carbs, hardly any fat, and no cholesterol or purine.

Seitan can be kept for three to four days in the fridge (in its stock) and for months in the freezer.

Cook it with the lid on the pan over a gentle heat and avoid searing it as this makes it go hard.

Even better, try cooking seitan in a frying pan as this softens it up even more. And to retain the texture and flavour, it's best to avoid using thick slices.

Mix together herbs, spices, garlic and soy sauce and dip your seitan into this marinade before frying it. Leave the seitan slices to soak up the sauce of your choice, and from Tuesdays onwards you can serve them with vegetables.

Tempeh
Another soy food product, originally from Indonesia, tempeh is made by fermenting soya beans. It has a firm texture and a natural flavour of hazelnuts and

mushrooms. High in protein, low in fat and with no cholesterol, tempeh is an ideal food for vegetarians.

Soya steaks or veggie burgers

As a vegetable alternative to meat, soya steaks or veggie burgers are essentially great for vegetarians. Usually they leave meat lovers dissatisfied, so they'll only try them when there's no other alternative. However, vegetarians enjoy eating them and, most importantly, they know best how to prepare them.

Always read the label to check the fat content, as some brands can contain double the normal amount – up to 8%, which is close to a semi-lean steak from the butcher's.

Textured soy protein

Textured soy – or vegetable (TVP) – protein comes in small granular chunks and looks like cereal. Made from soy flour, from which the oil has been removed, the flour is mixed with water and heated under pressure. The mixture is dried and either cut into small chunks or ground into granules.

There are many advantages to textured soy proteins. They contain twice as much protein as beef and are low in calories and cholesterol. Easy to store over a long period, they are also cheap and easy to cook with.

Once prepared, textured soy protein has a texture not dissimilar to meat, which allows vegetarians to enjoy dishes and recipes that traditionally use meat.

However, uncooked, this protein is also nice and crunchy with a slight natural taste of peanuts, making it a pleasant and handy snacking food.

Soy milk

A non-dairy drink that is high in vegetable proteins, low in calories, fats, calcium and vitamin D and devoid of cholesterol. For anyone who has to watch their cholesterol or who can't digest cow's milk (vegetarians, the lactose intolerant or anyone who simply dislikes the taste), soy milk provides a good substitute.

It comes plain and flavoured and can be used to make any sauce that uses milk, such as béchamel and hollandaise.

It can be stored for five to seven days in the fridge.

Soy milk is not an 'as much as you want' food. You may have one glass a day to replace skimmed cow's milk and provided it's plain and not flavoured.

Soy yoghurt

Made from soy milk, soy yoghurt has the same characteristics and offers an alternative for people who are lactose intolerant or have trouble digesting dairy products.

As far as nutrition and calories go, it's very similar to yoghurt made from semi-skimmed milk. Depending on the brand, the average fat content is around 2% and there's no cholesterol.

You can't eat as much soy yoghurt as you want; you must stick to two pots a day, and, of course, it has to be plain.

9. Fat-free Dairy Products (Yoghurt, Fromage Frais, Cottage Cheese and Quark)

Created to make slimming easier, these foods are proper dairy products and in all respects are just the same as traditional yoghurts, fromage frais and cottage cheese products except that the fat has been removed.

As processing milk into cheese is responsible for getting rid of lactose, the only sugar found in milk, these low-fat dairy products contain less of it and are therefore richer in proteins. For several years now, dairy-product manufacturers have been bringing out new generations of low-fat yoghurts that are sweetened, flavoured or have added fruit pulp. Whereas the sweeteners and flavourings are just calorie-free decoys, adding fruit does introduce a small but undesirable amount of carbs. Therefore, to be absolutely clear, there are three types of fat-free yoghurt: plain, flavoured – e.g. coconut, vanilla, lemon – and fat-free but fruity yoghurts i.e. those containing little bits of fruit or some compote at the bottom. Only plain and flavoured yoghurts are completely allowed without any restriction. So avoid all fruity yoghurts and, when you get to Wednesday, opt for fresh fruit instead.

10. 1.5 Litres (2½ Pints) of Liquid Per Day

This is the only category on the list that is compulsory; all the others are optional, so you just follow your own desires.

Drinking is a vital function and even more so if you're trying to slim down. However carefully you follow your diet, it's likely to stagnate if you don't drain your body thoroughly, as the waste by-products of burning up your fat will accumulate until you stop losing weight.

All types of waters are allowed, especially spring waters that are slightly diuretic. However, you should avoid Badoit and San Pellegrino, which are excellent but contain too much sodium.

If you dislike still water, then drink fizzy water instead – bubbles and gas have no impact whatsoever on this diet. Sodium is the one thing to avoid.

If you're not a fan of cold drinks, then remember that coffee, tea or any other infusion or herbal tea are akin to water and, as such, count towards the obligatory 1.5 litres (2½ pints). Finally, as a doctor and nutritionist, I've taken personal responsibility for allowing diet drinks such as Diet Coke or any other brand with only one calorie per glass. You will know that among the general public, and even among nutritionists, this is a hotly debated topic. Some think that our bodies can detect the deception and will compensate for it. Others maintain that these drinks encourage a need and taste for sugar.

As far as I'm concerned, what I've learnt from working with patients is that however long abstinence may last, it never eradicates our taste and need for sugar. So I can't see any reason why you should deprive yourself of this calorie-free flavour. Furthermore, I've seen how these drinks make it so much easier for people to stick to the diet. The sugary flavour, high aromatic content, colour and fizz, as well as the impression of being a party drink, all combine to make fizzy drinks a comfort food that provides a great sensory experience and calms those cravings for 'something else' that inveterate snackers so frequently experience when dieting.

Sweeteners are the subject of a different controversy. Some people claim they're carcinogenic and I quite understand how you might be worried by this. You need to remember that for over 50 years there has been a succession of different sweeteners and, with each new product, the same controversy flares up – which, to my mind, seems rather suspect. Let me remind you too that sweeteners are 'permitted' everywhere worldwide and, to my knowledge, not a single country has set any restrictions other than the maximum daily dose. Although billions of people use them daily, there hasn't been one single complaint from a consumer. Whereas, let me point this out again, being overweight, obesity and diabetes are amazing killing machines. And from observing it on a daily basis, I know personally that sweeteners make it far easier for us to tackle these terrible health problems. Why, as a matter of caution taken to absurd extremes, should we cast doubt on such fantastic tools, when they offer us taste and flavour but without the calories or insulin? That's my opinion. Of course you can do as you choose, but my wife, my children and I all use them regularly.

11. 1½ Tablespoons of Oat Bran Per Day

For years, the first two actual weight-loss phases in my method didn't include any starches, starchy foods or cereals.

This didn't stop it from working, but so many people who used it eventually ended up yearning for . . . carbs!

While I was attending a cardiology conference in New York I came across oat bran. This was at a time when America had declared war on cholesterol, as it was the country with the highest number of deaths from heart attacks.

In 1988, using studies based on very wide populations, American authors proved that oat bran reduced blood cholesterol content. This announcement was like a bomb going off and oat bran consumption exploded. In the 1990s oat bran muffins had their hour of glory and even made the front page of the *New York Times.*

Pharmaceutical laboratories then discovered fibrates and later statins, medication that is now used worldwide to treat cholesterol reliably and effectively, so oat bran was then forgotten about. In short, at this conference, a vegetarian cardiologist who was still attached to her oat bran gave me a packet that went home in my suitcase. One morning, my very hungry daughter Maya, unable to find anything she fancied in what she called a 'nutrition-ist's kitchen', asked me to help her make a snack. As we'd run out of flour, I concocted an improvised crêpe with some oat bran, fromage frais, an egg, a little cinnamon and some sweetener – because, I'll let you in on a secret, that will hardly come as a surprise, there's no white sugar in my home!

Maya was both delighted and felt full. At one o'clock she phoned me from her school canteen to say that oddly enough she didn't feel at all hungry and was worried about this. Was this down to her 'odd crêpe'? This is how it all started. So I recommended oat bran to some of my patients who were very big eaters and my initial hunch was confirmed. This is how oat bran gradually found its place among the founding principles of my method. In fact, in my original method it's the only carb admitted into the Attack phase's pure protein sanctuary.

From a clinical perspective, what I soon noticed was an overall improvement in results: it was easier to stick to the diet; appetite lessened; the feeling of being full came sooner and frustration decreased significantly over time.

Oat bran

Oat bran is the fibrous husk that surrounds and protects the oat grain. For a long time, only the grain and its mild texture were of any interest and oats were made into flour and rolled oats. Low-sugar, high-fibre oat bran was fed to animals and used to stuff mattresses and pillows.

To understand how oat bran works, I examined studies conducted by American cardiologists who proved that it reduced the absorption of intestinal cholesterol. Diabetes specialists observed how it slowed down the assimilation of fast sugars in the intestines. Naturally, this caught my attention, and I investigated further to see what happened as oat bran passed through the digestive tract, the stomach and then the small intestine.

I realized that its fibre had two physical properties that gave it a medicinal role:

Its ability to absorb: oat bran can absorb over 20 times its volume of water. To see this for yourself, you only need to test it out with a bowl and some water. Likewise, as soon as it reaches the stomach, oat bran swells up and takes up enough space to mechanically and rapidly make you feel full by simply distending your stomach.

It is extremely viscous: once it arrives in the small intestine, mixed in with food that has by now turned to pulp, the oat bran sticks to all the surrounding nutrients. By doing this, the bran stops them being absorbed into the blood and takes some away with it into the stools.

Since oat bran makes you feel full and helps you lose calories, it became a valuable ally in my battle against weight problems. It became integral to my original method and I prescribe it to you in this second front, starting with Monday, the day devoted to proteins.

However, do bear in mind that not all oat brans are equally good. Depending on the manufacturer, the milling and sifting (separating the flour and oat bran) can vary. According to my research, M2bis-B6 index oat bran is the best; it produces medium-sized particles and is sifted six times to lower the carb content. This means it has the best medicinal effects and the biggest impact on dieting. I have even written a short book about this foodstuff, *The Oat Bran Miracle*, because it really deserves your full attention. Oat bran is a food friend; stick with it and it'll never let you down.

How should you eat your oat bran?
As part of the second front, your daily dose is $1\frac{1}{2}$ tablespoons.

The savoury/sweet oat bran galette
(see recipe on page 143)
Galettes can be kept for up to a week in the fridge, wrapped in foil or in a plastic container to prevent them from going dry. You can also freeze them; they will retain their flavour, texture and goodness.

Most of my patients eat their galette in the morning, which prevents them from feeling famished mid-morning. Others eat their galette as a lunchtime sandwich with a generous slice of smoked salmon or bresaola.

There are others who eat a galette in the middle of the afternoon, when they are overcome by cravings and are in danger of 'sinning'. Some even have a galette after dinner, when they get the urge to go rummaging in cupboards to find something comforting before bedtime.

If you'd like to have a go at other oat bran recipes, you'll find lots for pancakes, muffins, pizza bases, gingerbread loaves and bread on the internet.

You'll find lots of products made with oat bran in the supermarkets, such as biscuits, snack bars and galettes, which you may eat as long as you don't exceed the recommended amount.

Check that these foods don't contain any refined wheat flour because, along with sugar, this is the greatest trigger for insulin secretion, which in turn produces fat. For an equal number of calories, these are the most fattening ingredients there are.

Another good thing about the oat bran galette is that it has proved to be a great tool for helping bulimics to control their cravings. A person who forces him or herself to throw up on a regular basis needs psychotherapeutic help to deal with what is a serious condition. However, if by chance any bulimics do read my book, then remember that by eating as many oat bran galettes as you want with whatever flavours you fancy, you can avoid the calorie spikes you get from eating other, poor quality foodstuffs. I've noticed this with my patients on a very regular basis.

Bulimic or not, you may still go through difficult periods in your life when you feel overcome by irresistible urges – so you give in and instantly you've undermined the time you've just spent watching your weight correctly! Should this happen, you may, over a short period, increase your oat bran intake and eat up to three galettes a day.

12. Konjac

Along with oat bran, konjac is the second food that to my great delight has become part of my work as a nutritionist. I'm convinced that in years to come it will play a major role in the worldwide fight against weight problems, obesity and diabetes.

As far as I'm concerned, konjac is not simply a food – it's a food concept, and it has arrived in the nick of time to protect modern man, whose life is endangered by exposure to such an over-abundance of food.

Konjac overturns the rule that says that the foods that most attract us are the ones highest in calories and carbs. Our ancestors living in the savannahs would have shunned konjac, but for our industrialized societies and for nutritional dieting this food is a godsend.

LET ME DESCRIBE THIS FOOD IN MORE DETAIL

Part of Japan's food heritage, konjac has been used for centuries. I came across it when I was eating in a restaurant there with my publisher. I tasted 'shiratakis', which look a bit like Chinese rice noodles. My publisher explained that they were made from konjac, a local vegetable. He told me how, as with all treasured foods, konjac has its own myth, a wonderful story about its origins – the Japanese believe that it's a gift from the gods. Every year they celebrate it with a day's festival.

When I returned home, I discovered by chance that konjac is a food devoid of calories, and therefore that the pasta I'd eaten was calorie-free. You can imagine my astonishment as a nutritionist at stumbling across such a bizarre thing as 'friendly pasta'! And my jubilation as a doctor fighting weight problems, obesity and diabetes at suddenly having at my disposal such a magical foodstuff!

Konjac is a plant root, the size of a large beetroot, which grows buried under the ground. When the season is right, a stem appears from the tuber; it grows and little branches, leaves and flowers then develop.

What is special about konjac is that it lives from the reserves held inside itself. Inevitably, the moment arrives when the plant has used up all its reserves and it shrivels up, withers and dies. The story could well end here, but the Japanese harvest the tubers, which are packed with a soluble fibre, glucomannan. The konjac tubers are ground into a powder that the Japanese then use to produce a whole range of food products. For centuries they had no idea that they were eating a food with no calories; they enjoyed it for its crisp, elastic consistency, a quality they also appreciate in seaweed and other vegetables unfamiliar to us in the West. In Japan, the most common konjac product is shirataki noodles. Many scientific works and studies have looked at konjac powder and analyzed its medicinal properties.

How konjac works
- It has a powerful effect on appetite, **making us feel full quickly** and then we feel satiated.
- It **reduces cholesterol and triglyceride levels**, and can be used to protect against cardiovascular pathologies.
- It has **a combined effect on sugar metabolism**, as the soluble fibre works away to slow down digestion and

assimilation of sugar and high glycaemic index carbs, such as white flour and starchy foods.

Since making these discoveries, I've been working hard to improve this food and make it more widely known, so that it becomes part of our modern Western diet. If you're obese or diabetic, it's now possible to eat 'pasta' and to eat as much as you want. Konjac is good for you because not only is it calorie-free, but it's packed with soluble fibre that helps to slow the passage of nutrients into the bloodstream. Could we ask for more?

Just as we now have diet fizzy drinks, sugar-free chewing gum and fat-free dairy products, I'm campaigning to spread the word about konjac, as a diet alternative to starches and starchy foods.

Nowadays, given our obesity and weight problem epidemic, we have to face the facts – as foods, pasta and white rice are simply too rich for us because they're almost entirely made up of medium-penetration carbs. Anything made with white flour puts the pancreas under too much strain, making it secrete insulin. Frequently served as an accompaniment, we consume these starchy foods in large quantities and often, thereby encouraging diabetes and the storage of fat due to the impact of their calories. This is one factor for sure that is producing more and more overweight people across the planet.

A really important fact to bear in mind is that, in Europe, the nation that eats the most konjac is Italy, the world's undisputed leader when it comes to pasta and its staunchest defender.

How should I eat my konjac?

First of all, you can CHOOSE how much you eat; as with all the other Monday foods there's no restriction. You'll stop when you feel full up and replete, which is what happens with this magical food.

There are many different ways in which it can be used but, given our European tastes, I recommend you try either pasta or rice.

Konjac pasta

Konjac pasta comes in different varieties.

The most traditional sort, which I initially advocated using, are konjac noodles. Since then I've been working closely with Asian manufacturers to come up with different shapes. Now you can buy konjac tagliatelle and spaghetti, and very soon penne, farfalle, linguine and fusilli will be available.

Monday's key recipe is tagliatelle with Bolognese sauce. Add some minced beef in tomato sauce to your konjac pasta – but only a little sauce, just for flavour, as it's not a vegetable here. Vegetables only appear on your Nutritional Staircase on the next day, i.e. on Tuesday.

You can enjoy your konjac pasta with some pesto and coriander, or with garlic, white wine vinegar and a little cayenne pepper. I'd also suggest adding strips of smoked salmon, small pieces of chicken, calf's liver, prawns, scallops, sliced sausage (grilled beforehand to cook out the fat) and low-fat ham or rindless bacon. And, most importantly, don't forget to use herbs and spices liberally because although konjac has no particular taste of its own, it absorbs any flavours with which it comes into contact. So you could try coriander, garlic, onion, pesto, curry powder, turmeric, cumin, paprika and even marinated ginger.

Konjac rice or tapioca

Available in health food and Asian stores, konjac rice allows you to introduce some variety into this second front. The rice has a very different texture to the pasta, as it tends to disappear as you bite into it. However, as there is so much in a mouthful this creates a rather pleasant friction, which helps to bring out the flavour you've added to it.

As with the pasta, you can prepare the rice in endless ways: for example, tabouleh, risotto in all its guises, and rice pudding with chocolate sauce (using either 1% fat cocoa powder or flavouring).

Cayenne Pepper

For a long time we've known about the thermogenic benefits of cayenne pepper, and this should be of interest to you now.

Thermogenesis takes place when the body produces heat by increasing cell metabolism. Under normal circumstances, this happens during many chemical processes that the body undergoes, such as digestion, assimilation, combustion and so on. Your body uses one of these thermogenic processes to keep itself above the minimum survival temperature.

To improve the results you can obtain with my diet, I've studied in great detail the role played by cold and adapting to the cold.

The principle is that of homeothermia, i.e. human body temperature has to be kept above 35.5 °C. To maintain this temperature, the body is prepared to burn all its calories just to survive.

If you take a bath or shower in water at a temperature below that of your body, you'll force your body to burn up calories so that it doesn't get dangerously cold and run the risk of hypothermia. When you swim in 20 °C water, and your body has to keep itself at 36–37 °C, it needs to 'warm itself up' a lot and fast, and in doing so it uses up far more calories than for your front crawl or breaststroke.

The same applies to what you drink. When you drink a bottle of water that has come out of the fridge at 4 °C and you eliminate this water as urine at 36 °C, you're forcing your body to burn enough calories to raise the temperature of the litre of water by 32 °C. It's the same heat, and therefore the same number of calories a stove would burn to do this work. You don't need to get bogged down in the calculations, as I've already worked out that it's a little over 50 calories.

So thermogenesis is about burning up calories. The organ that regulates your thermogenesis is your thyroid gland. Which explains why people with hypothyroid-ism, who don't produce enough of this hormone, generate less heat to warm themselves than others and they tend to feel the cold. If they eat and exercise just the same as other people, they'll still put on weight more easily and, if dieting, they'll have greater diffi-culty losing it.

As you know, foods are made up of a varying combina-tion of the three universal nutrients: proteins, fats and carbohydrates. I've already explained that the way in which food gets digested and then assimilated depends on the composition of these nutrients. Remember that this work is undemanding for fats and carbohydrates – requiring only two or three calories per 100 calories eaten. However, with proteins it takes a lot of work to dismantle the long chains of amino acids which are very firmly welded together. For every 100 calories eaten, 32 get burned up. Here again there is a difference in thermogen-esis, and proteins are very thermogenic.

So, you might ask, what does all this have to do with cayenne pepper? Well, cayenne pepper is a very strong spice that raises your body's basic level of thermogenesis and produces an effect similar to when we react to cold, break down proteins and take exercise. Only to a very marginal extent, of course, but it's still enough to be useful as part of a weight-loss programme.

What's more, it turns out that green tea has a similar, well-known effect, so much so that many laboratories use it to make so-called 'fat-burning' food supplements.

As part of this second front, Mondays are about eating proteins which have a thermogenic effect. So I'm also going to suggest you try making a drink specially designed to increase thermogenesis and improve your Monday results.

Monday's drink: green tea with cayenne pepper, an activating infusion

Make up an infusion with 15g (½oz) of green tea leaves or green tea pearls and 1 litre (1¾ pints) of water. Add a pinch of cayenne pepper, the juice of 1 small lime and 4 teaspoons of sucralose. And don't forget how important cold is for thermogenesis, so cool this infusion as much as possible before drinking it in five portions spread over the day.

Combined together, the **caffeine**, **capsaicin** in the pepper, **lime**, the **coldness** of the drink, your **proteins** and **walking** all help not only to increase your body's thermogenesis, but also to improve elimination from the kidneys, so that your body gets drained more effectively throughout the day on Mondays.

I'll say it again, and this repetition is my way of supporting you: have cold drinks and walk for as much time as you can spare to further boost the thermogenesis set in motion by eating your Monday proteins. And don't forget – I can never repeat this often enough either – water is the very best natural, mechanical appetite suppressant.

However, perhaps you have a hypersensitive stomach and can't tolerate spices, pepper or chilli. Well, if you can't try this infusion, simply drink water instead, lots of water.

Extras

- **Skimmed milk**, either fresh, UHT or powdered is allowed. With tea and coffee, it improves the flavour and consistency. It can also be used to make sauces, custards, creams and in all sorts of dishes incorporating the ingredients you're allowed such as fromage frais, sweeteners, agar-agar, reduced-fat cocoa etc.
- **Sweeteners** are permitted, sugar is banned. For anyone who doesn't wish to use synthetic sweeteners, I recommend stevia, which is completely natural. For anyone seeking a perfect taste as close as possible to sugar, I'd recommend sucralose; it's what I use myself.
- **Vinegar, seasoning and herbs** – thyme, garlic, parsley, onions, shallots, chives etc. can all be freely used.
- **Spices**, just like herbs, are not only allowed but are strongly recommended. They will enhance the flavour of foods and increase their sensory value, which means that the nerve centres controlling satiety register all the taste sensations while you're eating and this makes you feel fuller.

  Spices are not just taste enhancers, which would be quite good enough, but they also make losing weight easier. What some spices, such as vanilla or cinnamon, do is swap their warming, reassuring flavour for the sugary one.

Others, for example coriander, curry powder, Colombo powder and cloves, can reduce the need to eat something salty. This is especially useful for anyone with water retention who has trouble stopping themselves from adding salt to food before they've even tasted it.

Finally, I'd like to underline just how good cayenne pepper, ginger and wasabi are because of their thermogenic effect.

- **Gherkins**, as well as **onions**, are allowed on your Monday, but only if they're used as condiments and not if the amounts are such that they'd have to be categorized as vegetables.

- **Lemon** may be used to flavour fish and seafood but not for lemon juice drinks and lemonade, even without sugar, because the lemon is then no longer a condiment but a fruit – an acidic one to be sure, but fruit has to wait until Wednesday to make its appearance in your week.

- **Salt** and **mustard** are allowed but must be eaten in moderation, particularly if you suffer from water retention, which is often the case for teenagers with irregular periods, premenopausal women and women starting HRT treatment. If you can't do without these flavours, you can find reduced-sodium salts and salt-free mustards.

- Ordinary ketchup is not allowed as it is both very salty and very sweet. However, if you like adding ketchup to your meat, you can use **sugar-free diet ketchup**.

Chewing gum

Chewing gum deserves more than just a brief mention in the extras category. For me, it's an important weapon in fighting weight problems. I don't use it much myself, but I do have some whenever I'm feeling stressed.

'Bruxism' is the term given by dentists to the night-time condition of teeth grinding during sleep, to the point where the enamel is worn down. And since many overweight people eat 'under stress', chewing gum can reduce their reflex action to chew food when stressed. What's more, if your mouth is full of chewing gum, there's no room for anything else. Clearly, I'm talking here about sugar-free gum, which nowadays is tasty and available in a whole range of stimulating flavours.

Many scientific studies prove on a regular basis that chewing gum has a part to play in preventing weight problems, diabetes and tooth decay.

What should we think about the nutritional composition of sugar-free chewing gum and which should we choose?

Sugar-free actually means no table sugar or saccharose. Polyols are mostly used to sweeten chewing gum; they do contain calories but their sweetening power is so much greater than ordinary sugar that only a very tiny quantity is required. In addition, polyols are absorbed and then assimilated in the intestines very slowly, so insulin secretion isn't stimulated and fat isn't created to be stored away. Select sugar-free chewing gum according to taste, but go for the gum whose flavour lasts longest in your mouth.

So for your Monday, apart from these extras and the 12 main categories previously described, there is NOTHING ELSE.

Anything else, anything not expressly mentioned on this list is forbidden today. But remember that come Tuesday there'll be something new, and this will set the pattern for each day until Sunday.

Exercise

With this seven-day weight-loss programme, Monday is the most powerful day of the week. You need to follow Mondays to the letter. As far as expending energy goes, try to boost your results by adding a suitable dose of exercise. Your instructions are to be active while not making yourself either hungry or tired. Walking as much as possible is the best way to achieve this, and certainly you should walk for at least 20 minutes. An hour would be ideal, but I realize that few of you have the time and leisure. For those of you who are younger, a 20–30-minute jog would be a great idea. So remember this one requirement: walk for at least 20 minutes on Mondays!

A Few General Tips

Eat as often as you want
On Mondays you can eat as much as you wish and before you even start to feel hungry, as you need to do everything

you can to avoid giving in to the temptation of a food that's not on your list.

Never skip a meal

This would be a serious mistake, albeit motivated by good intentions – but, as you know, the road to hell is paved with good intentions. Skipping meals is likely to gradually compromise this short Monday, which is so important for the rest of your week. What you don't eat during one meal is merely a false economy, since it'll be offset immediately by eating more at your next meal and, even worse, your body will make sure it extracts every last calorie from this catch-up meal.

What's more, once your hunger has been aroused, it tends to go for the most comforting foods, this is how hunger works, which will force you to draw on even more willpower to resist. Putting yourself under this sort of strain too often can undermine even the most motivated dieter. So never skip a meal and eat plenty.

Every time you eat, have something to drink

For some strange reason, advice from the 1970s advocating that people shouldn't drink at mealtimes still persists in our thinking today. For the average person, this advice is of no use whatsoever, and can even prove harmful for those on a diet. Failing to drink while you eat means quite simply that you run the risk of forgetting to drink altogether. What's more, drinking while you eat increases the volume in your stomach, making you feel replete and satisfied. Lastly, water dilutes your food, slows down its absorption and leaves you feeling fuller for longer.

Never run out of the foods you need for Monday
Always have to hand or stocked in your fridge plenty of the 12 categories of foods. They're going to become your friends and your talisman foods. When you travel, take them with you. Most protein foods require some preparation, so think ahead to what you'll need. Unlike carbs and fats, proteins cannot be stored for as long and are not as likely to be found in cupboards or drawers as biscuits and chocolate.

Before you eat a food, make sure
it's on your Monday list
To avoid making mistakes, keep this list with you for the first few days. What you're allowed to eat on Monday you can have for the rest of the week too. And I'll go further and say for the rest of your life, and always with these magic words: 'as much as you want'.

Your 'as much as you want' food list for Monday:

- Lean meat and offal
- Fish and shellfish
- Poultry
- Lean cooked meats and eggs
- Vegetable proteins
- Fat-free dairy products
- Water

- A little oat bran
- Konjac

Breakfast

Nutritionally, it is far more satisfying, as well as filling and energizing, to eat high-protein foods for breakfast than a pastry or chocolate-coated cereal. You can have milk in your coffee and tea, sweetened with aspartame or not, and a yoghurt, a boiled egg or slice of low-fat cooked turkey.

Breakfast is an ideal time to make your oat bran galette. If you're in too much of a rush then you can mix your oat bran into some hot milk, sweetened with aspartame or not, to make a porridge. Alternatively, you can stir it into yoghurt, which gives it a cereal taste and greater thickness.

At the restaurant

The easiest thing for you would be to avoid restaurants altogether on Monday. This opening day is so important that it's really not the moment to be tempting the devil. However, if you do have to go out, don't fret – all you need to do is keep in mind all the foods you are allowed to have and you'll soon see that nobody will even notice that you're dieting, not even you!

Let's imagine you're in a restaurant. For your starter, you can choose from a nice egg dish, a large slice of smoked salmon or a seafood platter. Next you have a wide choice for your main course; for example, grilled sirloin, roast beef, a veal chop, Japanese-style raw fish or grilled fish, roasted chicken or chicken breast. And why not go for rabbit with mustard or calf's liver deglazed in vinegar? Enjoy your food and eat until you feel full.

The difficult part comes after the main course, as this is when the cheese lover or pudding fan is accustomed to finishing off a meal with a third course. So how do you put such temptations out of reach? From experience, the best defensive strategy is to order a coffee straightaway. If the conversation keeps flowing, you can always ask for a second cup. Another useful tip is to have some flavoured chewing gum, which allows you to finish off your meal with a tasty flourish. Some restaurants are starting to put low-fat and even fat-free dairy products on the menu, but they are few and far between. If this isn't on offer, keep some plain or flavoured yoghurt in your office or car to use whenever necessary. You see, it's not all that difficult, especially if you think ahead and plan what you can do.

On the first Monday, **weigh yourself really frequently**. It's quite possible that you will notice a change from hour to hour.

You should, in any case, stick to the habit of weighing yourself every single day. If the bathroom scales are the enemy of anyone putting on weight, they're the friend and just reward of someone who is losing it – and any weight loss, however tiny, will be the best way of boosting your motivation.

Do I need to take vitamins?

No, not at all. Not on this first Monday or on any of the other days that, week after week, will get you to your True Weight. You'll have no deficiencies of any kind throughout the programme, so there's absolutely no reason to take vitamin supplements.

Your Diet Summary Sheet for Monday

Today, the first Monday of your programme, you're allowed to feed yourself from the 12 food categories and the extras on the list below. Within these food categories, you'll be completely free to eat as you wish throughout the whole day.

So the key words are simple and non-negotiable: you can have everything that's on this list, you can have it all – but you cannot have anything that isn't on there.

- Lean meats: veal, beef (except rib of beef and rib-eye steak), grilled or roasted without any fat
- Offal: liver, kidneys, and calf's and beef tongue (the tip)
- All fish: oily, lean, white, cooked and uncooked
- All seafood (shellfish and crustaceans)
- All poultry, except goose and duck, and without any skin
- Low-fat, cooked, sliced ham, chicken and turkey
- Eggs
- Vegetable proteins

- Fat-free dairy products
- 1.5 litres (2½ pints) of water (low sodium)
- An oat bran galette or 1½ tablespoons oat bran in milk, yoghurt or fromage frais
- Konjac
- A compulsory 20-minute daily walk
- Your extras: coffee, tea, herbal teas, green tea with cayenne pepper, vinegars, seasonings, herbs, spices, gherkins, lemons (not lemon drinks), salt and mustard (in moderation)

AND NOTHING ELSE!

Tomorrow, Tuesday, you'll add another food group and this will continue until Sunday.

DAILY RECIPES

PURE PROTEIN RECIPES FOR *MONDAY*

(and the other days that follow too)

OAT BRAN GALETTE

(1 serving)
Preparation time: 3 minutes
Cooking time: 8–10 minutes

1½ tablespoons oat bran
1½ tablespoons fat-free fromage frais
1 egg

Combine all the ingredients until the mixture is smooth.

Warm a non-stick frying pan over a medium heat and pour in a quarter of the mixture. Leave to cook for about 4–5 minutes. Using a spatula, turn the galette over and cook it for a further 4–5 minutes. Repeat with the remaining mixture.

To make a lighter version, you can separate the egg white from the yolk. Beat the white until stiff and fold it in once you've made up the mixture.

For a sweet galette, try adding 1 tablespoon sweetener; and 1 teaspoon fat-reduced cocoa powder to make a

143

chocolate galette. For a savoury version, try adding a little salt to taste, or spices, flaked nori seaweed, fennel seeds, turmeric, a few sesame seeds and so on.

CHICKEN AND TURMERIC LOAF

(4 servings)
Preparation time: 10 minutes
Cooking time: 20 minutes

Turmeric is one of the healthiest spices there is, protecting us particularly against cancer and to some extent against diabetes. If you like the taste, use it as freely as you want.

8 eggs
1 pinch of ground coriander
1 pinch of turmeric
Juice of 2 lemons
2 chicken breasts, chopped into small pieces
Salt and black pepper

Preheat the oven to 180°C/350°F/Gas 4.

Hard-boil 2 of the eggs then peel and halve them. Break the remaining 6 eggs into a large bowl and beat them, adding salt, black pepper, the coriander, turmeric and half the lemon juice. Next, stir in the chicken pieces.

Lightly oil a round loaf tin then wipe it with some kitchen paper. Pour in the mixture and add the halved hard-boiled eggs.

Bake in the oven for about 20 minutes. Place a small container with 150–200ml (5–7fl oz) of water in the oven, to keep the loaf moist as it cooks. The loaf is ready once it is golden brown on top, but you can also check by inserting the tip of a knife.

Serve warm with the remaining lemon juice.

CRUSTY, SPICY TURKEY STRIPS

(4 servings)
Preparation time: 20 minutes + 2 hours marinating
Cooking time: 30 minutes

1 white onion, peeled and finely chopped
200g (7oz) virtually fat-free quark
1 tablespoon mustard
100g (3½oz) silken tofu
½ teaspoon French 4-spice mix (pepper, ground ginger, nutmeg and cloves)
Freshly ground black pepper
600g (1lb 5oz) turkey breast, cut into thin strips
A squeeze of lemon juice (optional)

Put the onion in a bowl and add the quark and mustard. Stir thoroughly to combine, then work in the silken tofu and spice mix. Season with freshly ground black pepper.

Add the turkey to the bowl and stir to coat with the quark mixture. Cover with cling film and place in the fridge for at least 2 hours (or, better still, overnight).

Preheat the oven to 200°C/400°F/Gas 6. Pour the turkey strips and marinade into an ovenproof dish and bake in the oven for 30 minutes. Turn them over several times while they are cooking.

Serve piping hot, drizzled with a squeeze of lemon juice, if liked.

SAUTÉED MEDITERRANEAN PRAWNS WITH CARAMELIZED GINGER

(4 servings)
Preparation time: 10 minutes
Cooking time: 5 minutes

For a long time Mediterranean prawns were an expensive food for special occasions. Like smoked salmon, they're now available to everyone, especially when frozen. If you like them, they're the

perfect food to eat during my diet's Attack phase:
they're one of the ten most filling foods that exist.

16 large, uncooked Mediterranean prawns, fresh or
frozen
1 small piece of fresh ginger, cut into thin strips
½ teaspoon powdered sweetener
½ teaspoon 5-spice powder
150g (5½oz) fat-free quark with garlic and fresh herbs

If the prawns are frozen, thaw them in the fridge on
some kitchen paper, then peel them carefully.

Warm a non-stick frying pan and add the ginger.
Next, add the sweetener, 5-spice powder and
prawns. Stir-fry them for 2–3 minutes over a fairly
high heat.

Deglaze the pan by melting the quark. Turn the heat
down as low as possible and simmer for 1 minute,
stirring very carefully. Serve immediately.

STEAK MARINATED IN BALSAMIC VINEGAR AND MUSTARD

(4 servings)
Preparation time: 15 minutes + at least 3 hours
marinating
Cooking time: 15 minutes

An excellent recipe that gives basic steak a festive air. Balsamic vinegar comes from Italy and has quickly become popular worldwide, and quite rightly so, as it has an extremely unusual taste. Combined with ginger and paprika, you either love it or you hate it. If you love it, you'll keep coming back to this recipe.

3 tablespoons balsamic vinegar
1 tablespoon soy sauce
2 tablespoons Dijon or wholegrain mustard
4 beef steaks
Salt and black pepper
Paprika, to taste
1 tablespoon finely chopped ginger, to serve

In a large, shallow dish, mix together the vinegar, soy sauce and mustard.

Add the steaks to the dish and cover with cling film. Refrigerate for at least 3 hours (or, better still, overnight). Turn the steaks over at least once.

Remove the steaks from the fridge and place them on a wooden chopping board. Season to taste with some freshly ground black pepper and paprika.

Preheat the grill. Grill the steaks – try to keep them nice and juicy – for about 15 minutes, turning them halfway through. When cooked to your liking, serve the steaks sprinkled with the chopped ginger and some salt and black pepper.

MOROCCAN-STYLE MUSSELS

(4 servings)
Preparation time: 15 minutes
Cooking time: 15 minutes

Did you know that fossilized mussel shells have been found on many prehistoric archaeological excavation sites? Proof that our ancestors, the hunter-gatherers, enjoyed them long ago too!

2 litres (3½ pints) mussels
2 carrots, finely sliced
2cm (¾in) piece of fresh ginger, finely sliced
4 shallots, finely chopped
2 garlic cloves, finely chopped
½ bunch of fresh coriander, finely chopped
½ bunch of fresh parsley, finely chopped
1 teaspoon paprika
1 teaspoon cumin seeds
1 preserved lemon, finely chopped
Juice of 1 lemon
Salt and black pepper

Wash and scrub the mussels. Place them in a large bowl and with water. Swirl them around and replace the water. Do this several times until the water is quite clean and there are no half-opened or broken mussels floating on top. Drain well.

In a large saucepan with a little water added, cook the carrots, ginger, shallots, garlic, half the chopped coriander and parsley, paprika, cumin seeds, preserved lemon and some salt for 10 minutes over a gentle heat.

Next add the mussels and lemon juice to the pan and stir. Cook for a few minutes until all the mussels have opened up (discard any that refuse to open).

Serve the mussels nice and hot with some black pepper and the rest of the coriander and parsley.

VEAL WITH THYME AND LEMON

(4 servings)
Preparation time: 10 minutes marinating
Cooking time: 5 minutes

4 thin slices of veal
1 bunch of lemon thyme
Juice of 3 lemons

2 tablespoons cottage cheese
Salt and pepper

Cut the veal slices into thin strips.

Arrange the veal strips on a bed of lemon thyme in a baking pan, pressing down firmly. Mix until well covered and allow to stand for ten minutes.

Squeeze over the lemon juice.

Heat a non-stick frying pan over a high heat. Fry the veal slices for about 5 minutes, until golden brown. Season with salt and pepper and remove from the pan. Pour the lemon juice into the pan to loosen any cooking juices and add two tablespoons of cottage cheese to the sauce.

Return the veal to the sauce and let it reduce for about 1 minute. Serve piping hot.

Tuesday

THE LEITMOTIF
Monday for what's vital
Tuesday for what's essential
Wednesday for what's important
Thursday for what's useful
Friday for what's smooth and creamy
Saturday for energy
and Sunday for freedom!

Here you are, ready to place your foot on the second step of the Nutritional Staircase – the basic weekly programme for my second front. As you climb up its steps, remember that each day of the week will bring you something new and its own reward.

If you followed my instructions to the letter yesterday, you're bound to have lost some weight. How much? This will all depend on the total amount you have to lose, i.e. the difference between your starting weight and your True Weight. (Reminder: you can calculate this for free on my coaching website **www.regimedukan.com**)

If you're a man and have around 1½ stone to lose, you may well have shed a couple of pounds. This will depend on your weight background and the previous diets you've tried. If you've got 2¼ stone to lose, then you may have lost about 3 pounds. And if you've got just over a stone to lose, then reckon on around 1½ pounds.

If you're a woman then other parameters, such as age and hormonal balance (periods, contraception etc.) come into play. But if all is pretty calm, you'll have shed a couple of pounds if you're aiming to lose 1½ stone; or if it's more like a stone and a bit, 1½ pounds. Below that amount, it's hard to predict, but at any rate you'll have still lost over a pound.

Yesterday, I promised you that there would be something new today and here you go – the large, very large, vegetable family. You see, I wasn't having you on. From now on, in addition to your Monday protein foods, you're allowed all vegetables, cooked and uncooked; and once again there's absolutely no restriction on amount, time of day or combination.

So within your reach you now have: tomatoes, cucumber, radishes, spinach, asparagus, green beans, fennel, cabbage, mushrooms, celery, all types of salad, chard, aubergines, courgettes, peppers and even hearts of palm.

Please note, though, that you're not allowed any starchy foods – they'll come later. For the time being, leave potatoes, rice, sweetcorn, fresh or dried peas, chickpeas, split peas, broad beans, lentils and kidney beans well alone. Also forget about avocados: often thought to be a green vegetable, they are in fact a fruit and a high-fat, oleaginous one at that.

And to get the very best results, avoid carrots and beetroot as well as artichokes and salsify.

Also, rhubarb is the only 'fruit' allowed on Tuesdays. Why? Simply because rhubarb is not really a fruit at all and belongs to the vegetable family!

How Should I Prepare These Vegetables?

Uncooked vegetables: if you can tolerate and digest raw vegetables, it's always preferable to eat them when they're totally fresh and uncooked to avoid losing any of the vitamins.

THE PROBLEM WITH DRESSINGS

Despite appearing harmless, dressings pose one of the biggest problems for weight-loss dieting. For many people, salads and crudités are the quintessential diet food, low in calories, high in fibre and vitamins. This is absolutely correct, except that the dressing that comes with them can totally undermine this virtuous combination. To give you a simple example: take an ordinary salad bowl containing 2 large lettuces and 2 tablespoons of oil – the salad accounts for 20 calories and the oil for 280! These calories sneak their way in so craftily, which explains why so many diets based on mixed salads fail because they don't bother to check the calories contained in the dressings.

So the instruction is very simple, here's how you can prepare a risk-free dressing:

Maya Salad Dressing

Take an old mustard jar and fill it with the following ingredients:

1 tablespoon Dijon or grainy mustard
10 tablespoons balsamic vinegar
6 tablespoons sparkling water
1 teaspoon oil of your choice
8 basil leaves
If you like garlic, add a large uncrushed clove, just for taste.

Mix the ingredients thoroughly and then leave to infuse. Shake well before use.

It's a pity if you don't like balsamic vinegar, because it has the strongest sensory appeal. However, you can choose a different sort provided you add a little less: 4 tablespoons for wine, raspberry and sherry vinegar; and 3 tablespoons for spirit vinegar.

Did you realize that vinegar is a condiment that can play a major role in any weight-loss diet? It was discovered recently that man can distinguish four universal flavours – sweet, salty, bitter and sour. However, vinegar is the only substance on our human food list that provides this rare and precious sour taste, so don't hold back on the vinegar!

Furthermore, recent studies have also proven the positive impact of oral sensations; the quantity and variety of different flavours helps to produce feelings of satisfaction and fullness.

For example, it's been established that certain spices with intense flavours, such as cloves, ginger, star anise and cardamom encourage the accumulation of powerful, penetrating sensations that are able to increase the gauge in the hypothalamus, the area in our brains responsible for measuring these sensations, until the feeling of satiety is triggered. So it's very important to use the whole range of spices as widely and often as possible, and preferably at the start of a meal. So try and get used to them if you're not a diehard fan already.

If you tend to get constipated, or if this happens occasionally, replace vegetable oil with a mineral oil, for example paraffin oil, which is the world's oldest intestinal lubricant.

While we're on the subject of sauces, I'd like to take the opportunity here to clear up the ambiguity surrounding olive oil. Very often, when I ask my patients whether they use any oil, I get the answer: 'No, Doctor, only olive oil.'

Please be aware that although olive oil, a symbol of Mediterranean culture and cuisine, is unanimously acknowledged as the benchmark when it comes to protecting against cardiovascular disease, it is still nonetheless an oil and it contains just as many calories as any other oil. This means 9 calories per gram; and, by way of comparison, carbs have only 4 calories and proteins slightly fewer.

For anyone who doesn't like either vinegar or traditional dressings, it's possible to make a natural, flavoursome dressing using low-fat dairy products.

Low-fat natural yoghurt or fromage frais dressing
Choose low-fat natural yoghurt, which is a little creamier than the fat-free variety but has scarcely any more calories. Add 1 level tablespoon Dijon mustard to the yoghurt or fromage frais and beat together, whipping the mixture until it starts to thicken and resemble mayonnaise. Then add a dash of vinegar, season with salt and black pepper, sprinkle over some fresh herbs and enjoy!

Vegetables as a cooked accompaniment: now is the time to use those green beans, spinach, leeks, cabbage of all varieties, mushrooms, braised chicory, fennel, celery and so on.

You can cook these vegetables in water, boil them, or better still steam them to preserve as far as possible their taste and vitamin content.

You can also bake them in the oven in the juice from your meat or fish – think of classic dishes such as sea bass with fennel, sea bream with tomatoes, and cabbage stuffed with minced meat.

You should also consider cooking your vegetables 'en papillote', i.e. wrapped in foil, as this combines all the advantages as far as taste and nutritional value are concerned. It is a particularly good way of cooking fish – salmon, for example, remains tender when cooked on a bed of leeks or chopped aubergines.

A real treat is to eat your vegetables grilled or barbe-cued. You can use a ridged chargrill pan or a heavy-based non-stick frying pan if you don't have a grill on your oven.

It was in Spain that I started grilling and eating my vegetables this way; there they have sweet onions as large as sometimes the best Cantaloupe melons. Just imagine a plate of these melt-in-your-mouth onions, sliced and served with a few tomato halves, some sliced chicory and devilishly succulent sliced aubergine, finished off with a few slightly firmer chunks of courgette. Completely scrumptious!

It's when I'm relishing these flavours in moments like this that I like to think back to our great ancestors, the hunter-gatherers. For 90 per cent of the time our species has been in existence, man lived just as you're preparing to do this Tuesday. I'm being quite serious now; the vast majority of people from whom we today have evolved ate high-protein foods *whenever they could* – meat that they had to hunt in groups, fish they caught, birds and eggs they pinched whenever possible. Finding this food meant they had to walk almost six hours a day!

The women did the gathering; this usually entailed searching for vegetables, wild leaves, salad, bamboo leaves, wild fennel and many other different types of plant, depending on the climate and geography.

Was this all they had? I'd be lying to you if I stopped here. Twice a year in temperate climates there would be a season of fruit and grasses (graminae). But don't imagine it was anything like our artificially cultivated fruit, packed with sweet sap. Pollen studies have shown that the fruit of old was small, scrawny and fibrous, like the wild blackberries, gooseberries, blueberries and blackcurrants we find nowadays. What's more, seasons were very short and the birds always got the first pick.

And it was exactly the same with the wild grasses, such as emmer wheat, spelt or wild barley. I'm telling you all this to point out that on this Tuesday, at the start of your week, you already have possession of the foods that are fundamental to the human race. So, you see, it's a good start – fast and strong.

Adding vegetables on Tuesday introduces freshness and variety to Monday's food. It makes the programme easier and more comfortable. From now on, a great way to start your meals is with a well-seasoned salad, full of colour and flavour, or a hearty vegetable soup on winter evenings. You can then move on to your main course of fish or meat cooked slowly over flavourful, seasoned vegetables.

How Much Am I Allowed?

As I've said, there's no restriction on quantity. However, I would advise you to keep within the bounds of common sense. I know some patients who settle down in front of huge great platters of mixed salad and chomp away without actually feeling in the slightest bit hungry. Try to avoid this temptation, because vegetables are not entirely innocuous. So eat them only until your hunger is completely satisfied, and stop there. In no way does this alter the principle at the heart of my philosophy, and therefore by extension at the heart of my method, which is that there is no restriction on quantity. Whatever the amount of vegetables you ingest, you will carry on losing weight but at a less steady rate, especially at the beginning. So just be sensible.

Can I Buy Ready Meals?

You see all sorts of ready meals on sale in supermarkets everywhere. Some purport to be health foods, with a proper nutritional balance, and consequently an aid to slimming. Once again, such claims are based on the calorie content.

If you want to be in tune with what my second front prescribes, forget about counting calories. It's a concept from the past which has done so much to scupper the fight against weight problems.

Start by checking the carbohydrate content of these ready meals. Carbs come in starchy foods such as potatoes, white rice, couscous and mashed potato. Cooked and then re-cooked, these starchy foods have a high glycaemic index. The glycaemic index, which we hear so much about, measures the extent to which high-carb foods will 'invade'.

What does 'invade' mean?

We're talking about the speed with which a food you've placed in your mouth enters your bloodstream. So why talk about 'invading'? How can this be harmful or even dangerous for your weight and health? It's quite simple: your body views these carbs, which arrive en masse and so quickly, as violent poisons. They could kill you. Your body defends itself, forced to react to them. For the time being, this saves your life but it makes you put on weight. If your pancreas didn't secrete insulin, half a loaf of bread could send you into a diabetic coma. However, this insulin only manages to rescue you by transforming the sugar into fat – and you know what happens next.

If you do want to buy ready meals, this is why you should avoid any that contain starchy foods until you get to Saturday.

So, if these ready meals are meant to be geared towards weight control, why do food manufacturers add these starchy foods, which we all know make us fat? Who stands to gain from this? The answer, again, is very simple: potatoes and rice are far less expensive than green vegetables. I'll keep on telling you this over and over again – sugars (carbs) should be seen as THE main reason why you have weight problems. I'll go even further:

If we cut down on carbs worldwide, by simply dropping the recommended 55–60 per cent daily amount to 25–30 per cent – which for people with a sedentary lifestyle is still a lot of energy – within 20 years there would be hardly any weight problems anywhere.

To come back to our ready meals, read the labels very carefully and note the protein content. Let's take as an example Asian pork and rice, a meal commonly found in supermarkets. You'll find almost 19% cooked, thinly sliced pork as opposed to around 47% Cantonese rice, the rest being water, pineapple, carrots, wheat flour, corn starch, etc. Why is there so little pork, so little animal protein in a meal that calls itself 'Pork and rice'? The reason is clear: animal protein costs a lot more than starchy foods. Meat and vegetables are far more expensive than pasta, potatoes, beans and rice. Always the same refrain! This allows the food-processing industry to reap substantial profits. Given how few 'good' products go into these ready meals (a kilo of Thai rice costs only a few pence!) they aren't such a cheap deal for us as we'd like to think.

So if you want to follow my second front by occasionally buying a few ready meals, select ones without starchy foods and that have as little fat as possible. You'll soon discover that they're not that easy to find . . .

Oat Bran

On Tuesday, stick to the same amount laid down for Monday, i.e. 1½ tablespoons, which is what you need to make your oat bran galette.

Tuesday's Drink: Green Tea with Cayenne Pepper

On Tuesday, carry on as you did yesterday and make your infusion with the same ingredients in the following quantities: 15g (½oz) green tea leaves or green tea pearls to 1 litre (1¾ pints) of water, a pinch of cayenne pepper, the juice of ½ lime and 2 teaspoons of sucralose.

Drink it nice and cold, divided between your two main meals, 500ml (18fl oz) each time.

Konjac

Your instruction remains and will always remain the same: complete freedom and variety. Don't be like my patient who stuck to eating ready-made konjac shirataki noodles with Bolognese sauce for both lunch and supper every single day. Enjoy a bit of variety, stimulate your taste buds and try out some new recipes – you'll find plenty on www.regimedukan.com and on internet forums. Konjac offers you a fantastic way to lose weight more easily. If it becomes a part of your eating habits, you'll stand a far better chance of not putting any weight back on. Konjac is your ally, so make it a food you enjoy too.

Exercise

Today your minimum amount is not a 20-minute walk but a **30-minute walk**. I'll keep stressing this over and over again – the more you walk, the better your results will be.

And I'm not recommending that you take exercise simply because it's a good way to burn up calories. There's another reason, which is even more important and has more impact on weight loss.

When exercise is adequate and regular – for example, 25 minutes every morning over more than four days – your brain will produce serotonin. And, as we've already seen, serotonin gives us a feeling of fulfilment. Deep down it works on life's pulsar by recharging it, so that inside you it maintains your need and desire to live – when this is a passing effect we tend to call it feeling on form and when it's permanent, happiness.

Don't ask me to say that happiness is just about exercising, as that would be far too simplistic. The happiness we're all looking for is based on ten things that generate well-being, what I refer to as the 'ten pillars of happiness', and exercise is only one of them.

The three most important sources of our vital energy are sexuality, food and social recognition.

So when a person decides to be more careful with their food intake, any extra serotonin produced by a daily walk is a very welcome boost and really helps things along.

I'd like to suggest a simple experiment to demonstrate to you just how true this is. On a day when you're feeling a bit down in the dumps and miserable, instead of dwelling on what's wrong, get out of the house and go for a run or a walk or a swim. And really give it your all, run at a good pace or walk briskly if you prefer walking. Take deep breaths and don't think about anything other than your body as it moves. This will take you half an hour at most and you'll be surprised by the results. Because you'll return home from your little excursion feeling much better and more optimistic, confident and cheerful. This is what I've been doing for the past 20 years and I can assure you that it keeps my morale rock solid. Give it a go yourself, as it's difficult to imagine how such a modest effort can have such a powerful impact on the brain and make it produce serotonin, a good mood and reasons to want to be alive.

An Important Question:
What Should I Do If I 'Slip Up'?

You've let yourself be tempted by friends or there's been some catastrophe or other incident and you've broken our contract. Don't panic. The next day, in this case Wednesday – or in general the day after the one when this happens – just revert to your Monday mode and have a high-protein-foods-only day. This will counterbalance any lapse.

I've devised this second front so that it works as effectively as possible while combining great flexibility and your gradual freedom to have as many foods as possible. My answer works for whichever day you're dealing with and will do so until you've lost your first 10 pounds.

Once you reach this stage and have lost that amount, your mission is half accomplished. As for the other half, it's up to you to decide if you want to persevere right to the end at my speed, or whether you want to take a little more time over it. However, I do advise you – and this advice is based on my experience with this second front – to FINISH while you're still up for it since 'a door should either be open or closed'!

Your Diet Summary Sheet for Tuesday

Today, on the first Tuesday of your programme, you're allowed Monday's 12 food categories **and Tuesday's vegetables**.

You can eat these vegetables without any restriction on quantity or time of day. However, be careful with dressings: try my Maya salad dressing or natural yoghurt dressing recipes instead.

- Lean meats: veal, beef (except rib of beef and rib-eye steak), grilled or roasted without any fat
- Offal: liver, kidneys, and calf's and beef tongue (the tip)
- All fish: oily, lean, white, cooked and uncooked
- All seafood (shellfish and crustaceans)
- All poultry, except goose and duck, and without any skin
- Low-fat, cooked, sliced ham, chicken and turkey
- Eggs
- Vegetable proteins
- Fat-free dairy products
- 1.5 litres (2½ pints) of water (low sodium)
- An oat bran galette or 1½ tablespoons oat bran in milk, yoghurt or fromage frais
- Konjac
- A compulsory 30-minute daily walk
- Your extras: coffee, tea, herbal teas, green tea with cayenne pepper, vinegars, seasonings, herbs, spices, gherkins, lemons (not lemon drinks), salt and mustard (in moderation)
- All cooked and uncooked vegetables

AND NOTHING ELSE!

DAILY RECIPES

PROTEIN AND VEGETABLE RECIPES FOR **TUESDAY**

(and the other days that follow too)

PORCINI MUSHROOM VELOUTÉ

(4 servings)
Preparation time: 10 minutes
Cooking time: 20 minutes

1 litre (1¾ pints) chicken stock, made from a stock cube
40g (1½oz) dried porcini mushrooms
200g (7oz) silken tofu
200g (7oz) virtually fat-free quark
Salt and black pepper
A few sprigs of chervil, finely chopped, to serve

In a saucepan, bring the stock to the boil with the dried porcini mushrooms and leave to reduce for 15 minutes. Sieve and set the stock aside.

Blend the mushrooms in a food processor with the tofu, quark and seasoning, then work the mushroom mixture into the stock.

Return to the saucepan and heat through. Leave the soup to reduce further over a gentle heat for 5 minutes.

Divide the soup among warmed serving bowls and serve sprinkled with the chervil.

TWO TOMATO TORTILLA

(4 servings)
Preparation time: 10 minutes
Cooking time: 20 minutes

1 shallot, finely chopped
8 eggs
100g (3½oz) fat-free fromage frais
8 sprigs of fresh basil, finely chopped
300g (10½oz) sundried tomatoes, cut into small pieces
150g (5½oz) cherry tomatoes, halved
Salt and black pepper
Salad leaves, to serve

Warm a non-stick frying pan over a gentle heat and add the shallot. Cover with a little water, season with salt and cook for about 5 minutes, until all the water has evaporated. Set aside.

Preheat the oven to 180°C/350°F/Gas 4.
Break the eggs into a large bowl and whisk them together. Beat in the fromage frais and basil, and season with salt and black pepper.

Arrange the dried tomatoes, cherry tomatoes and shallot in a flan dish, pour the egg mixture over them and bake in the oven for 15–20 minutes. Halfway through, cover the dish with some foil.

Serve the tortilla with a nice green salad.

ASPARAGUS AND BRESAOLA ROLLS WITH A HERB SALAD

(4 servings)
Preparation time: 15 minutes
Cooking time: 4 minutes

As well as being delicious, this dish has a high nutritional value.

20 green asparagus spears, trimmed
Mixed salad leaves (e.g. rocket, chervil, lamb's lettuce)
8 sprigs of parsley, finely chopped
8 sprigs of mint, finely chopped
8 sprigs of fresh coriander, finely chopped
20 slices of bresaola
50g (1¾oz) chives
1 tablespoon balsamic vinegar
4 tablespoons fat-free fromage frais
Salt and black pepper

Cook the asparagus in boiling water for 4 minutes. The spears should still be firm. Drain them on kitchen paper.

Prepare the salad by mixing together the leaves of your choice with the parsley, mint and coriander. Arrange the salad on 4 plates.

Roll each asparagus spear in a slice of bresaola with some chives, and place 5 asparagus rolls on each plate.

Make a dressing by combining the balsamic vinegar, fromage frais and seasoning. Serve with the rolls and salad.

KONJAC SHIRATAKI NOODLES WITH BOLOGNESE SAUCE

(2 servings)
Preparation time: 10 minutes
Cooking time: 1 hour minimum

1 garlic clove, finely chopped
1 onion, diced
1 carrot, finely diced
1 celery stick, finely chopped
Herbs: oregano, thyme, bay leaf
300g (10½oz) lean minced beef

1 jar of Dukan Diet tomato and coriander sauce (or 2 large tomatoes, peeled and roughly chopped)
250ml (9fl oz) low-salt beef stock
2 packets of Dukan Diet konjac shirataki noodles
Salt and black pepper

Place a large saucepan over a gentle heat and pour some water in the bottom. Add the garlic and onion and let them soften.

After a minute, add the carrot, celery, herbs, salt and black pepper and leave to cook for about 10 minutes. Add the minced beef, separating it out so that there are no lumps, and pour in the tomato and coriander sauce (or chopped tomatoes) along with the stock. Bring to the boil, check the seasoning and leave to simmer for 1 hour.

When the sauce is almost ready, rinse the konjac shirataki noodles in plenty of cold water. Bring a large pan of water to the boil, add the noodles and cook them for 2–3 minutes. Drain the noodles and rinse them in plenty of cold water.

Add the konjac shirataki noodles to the Bolognese sauce and serve piping hot.

Variation: You can replace the minced beef with 300g (10½oz) fresh salmon, cut into small pieces, and the tomato sauce with 8 tablespoons of fat-free fromage frais. Leave out the carrot and use dill instead of the other fresh herbs.

KONJAC TAGLIATELLE CARBONARA

(4 servings)
Preparation time: 10 minutes
Cooking time: 12 minutes

200g (7oz) extra-lean ham, cut into thin strips
4 tablespoons low-fat crème fraîche
2 packets of konjac tagliatelle
4 egg yolks
Salt and black pepper

Fry the ham in a non-stick frying pan for about 5 minutes. Add the crème fraîche and leave to simmer for 3 minutes. Season with salt and black pepper.

Meanwhile, rinse the konjac tagliatelle in plenty of cold water. Bring a large saucepan of lightly salted water to the boil, add the konjac tagliatelle and cook for 2 minutes. Rinse and drain the tagliatelle thoroughly then stir into the ham mixture in the frying pan. Leave to simmer for 2 minutes.

Divide the carbonara between 4 plates, carefully placing a whole egg yolk on top before serving.

VEGETABLE TARTARE WITH CHOPPED SMOKED SALMON

(4 servings)
Preparation time: 15 minutes
No cooking required

1 tablespoon mustard
2 tablespoons fat-free fromage frais
2 tablespoons cider vinegar
2 tablespoons balsamic vinegar
2 tomatoes, deseeded and finely diced
100g (3½oz) black winter radish, peeled and finely diced
50g (1¾oz) cucumber, finely diced
½ red pepper, finely diced
8 sprigs of dill, finely chopped
8 sprigs of chervil, finely chopped
2 slices of smoked salmon, finely diced
A few pink peppercorns
8 cos or other lettuce leaves
Salt and black pepper

Whisk together the mustard, fromage frais, both vinegars and add some salt and black pepper. Stir the vegetables and half of the herbs into this dressing.

Divide the mixture between 4 plates or dishes and sprinkle the smoked salmon over the top, followed by a few pink peppercorns.

Decorate each plate with two lettuce leaves and garnish with the remaining herbs.

DUKAN NEAPOLITAN PIZZA

(1 serving)
Preparation time: 10 minutes
Cooking time: 15 minutes

Here's a nice example of a diet recipe that the whole family can share. This Dukan pizza will be enjoyed by young and old alike, so forget about frozen pizzas!

Oat Bran Galette (see page 143), for the base
I garlic clove, finely chopped
500ml jar tomato passata
5 anchovy fillets
2 tablespoons capers
Oregano, fresh or dried
2 tablespoons low-fat cream cheese
1 pinch of cayenne pepper
Freshly ground black pepper

Use the oat bran galette recipe for the pizza base (see page 143).

Preheat the oven to 180°C/350°F/Gas 4. Mix the garlic and passata together then spread over the galette. Wipe away any oil from the anchovy fillets and arrange them on top. Scatter over the capers and oregano, and place little knobs of cream cheese all over the pizza. Add a pinch of cayenne pepper and season with a little black pepper.

Bake in the oven for 15 minutes.

RHUBARB MERINGUE COMPOTE

(4 servings)
Preparation time: 30 minutes
Cooking time: 30 minutes

Both a fruit and a vegetable, rhubarb is packed with vitamin C, potassium and phosphorus. As it's so high in fibre, it's a great food to eat as part of a diet.

600g (1lb 5oz) rhubarb, fresh or frozen
6 tablespoons crystallized stevia (or more according to taste)
Vanilla powder or vanilla flavouring
3 egg whites

3 tablespoons sweetener, suitable for cooking
1 pinch of salt

Rinse the rhubarb stalks and, without peeling them, chop into small 2–3cm (¾–1¼in) chunks. Place the rhubarb chunks in a saucepan and sprinkle over the crystallized stevia. Leave the rhubarb to release its juice for 10–15 minutes.

Cook the rhubarb in its own liquid over a gentle heat, taking care to stir at regular intervals. If necessary, add a little water. Add the vanilla powder or flavouring. Simmer for 30 minutes, until you have the compote consistency you want. Leave it to cool down.

Meanwhile, beat the egg whites until stiff with 1 tablespoon of the sweetener suitable for cooking and the salt. Once they are stiff, fold in the remaining sweetener and whisk for a further 15–20 seconds.

Divide the compote between 4 ovenproof ramekin dishes. Spoon the meringue on to each ramekin and heat under the grill for 10 seconds.

Wednesday

THE LEITMOTIF
Monday for what's vital
Tuesday for what's essential
Wednesday for what's important
Thursday for what's useful
Friday for what's smooth and creamy
Saturday for energy
and Sunday for freedom!

Here we are now on the third step as our journey continues; follow me as you're on the right track. Before I go into greater detail about what Wednesday involves, I'd like to digress for a moment. I get criticized for repeating the same messages too often. And I do indeed repeat things, but I do it on purpose. I've taught a lot of students, given explanations to many patients and written enough books to know that if you only say something once there's very little chance that it will be taken in or understood, and even less likelihood of it being remembered. All teachers and education experts agree with me. And if you feel aggrieved by my repeating myself then that means you've noticed it and that you've remembered a little, and maybe even a lot, of what I want to tell you.

Would you like an example?

When I say or write that you're allowed 'one celebration meal a week', far too often there have been patients who, in good faith, hear or read 'one celebration day'! When I say 'eat whichever green vegetables you want', some people straightaway include avocado, which is actually a fruit. And, even though they're detailed and precise, it's even worse when it comes to my instructions, which are passed on from person to person, from website to website and from country to country. This forces me to be vigilant and keep repeating my message to ensure that it's understood correctly.

End of digression.

So it's Wednesday today and the week is divided into three sections for our weight-loss programme:

1. **A section specifically for losing weight**, which covers the first four days – from Monday to Thursday. Monday is its spearhead; the loss continues on Tuesday and Wednesday but slows down gradually by Thursday.
2. **The second section** is Friday, which is the pivotal day. Weight loss stops but without opening the way for any weight gain. This is the day when your weight is held in balance.

3. **The third section** covers the weekend, Saturday and Sunday. Over these two days, your weight may increase slightly, but this will all depend on how you use your freedom. We'll go into this in greater detail once we've reached these steps on the Nutritional Staircase.

Before moving on to Wednesday's instruction, I'll remind you, as a leitmotif, what this second-front week is based on: Monday to Sunday, each new day brings you a food group, starting with what's most nutritional and ending with what's most comforting.

Today we're still in the weight-loss section of the week.

On Wednesday, you can treasure Monday's high-protein foods, still in unlimited quantities, along with all the Tuesday vegetables, also unlimited, and eat until you no longer feel hungry.

AND TODAY YOU ADD ONE FRUIT

Which one? Any, except bananas, grapes, dried fruit such as dried apricots and prunes, and oleaginous fruits like walnuts, almonds, peanuts, pistachios and other nuts.

Say no to tinned fruit in syrup, but yes to frozen fruit. And yes to fruit compote if it has 'no added sugar' – please check the labels carefully.

So you do have some choice, but fruit is allowed only if you associate it with the idea of portion control:

1 bowl of strawberries or raspberries

1 medium orange or 2 mandarins

2 figs

2 medium-sized kiwis

1 medium-to-large apple

1 medium-to-large pear

1 slice of fresh pineapple, 2cm (¾in) thick

½ medium-sized Charentais melon

1 slice of watermelon

½ mango or papaya, cut right down to the seed

And yes to rhubarb compote, home-made or shop-bought if you can manage to find it with no added sugar. There is no restriction on quantity: rhubarb is the only fruit you're allowed to have as much as you want of, but only provided you don't add any other fruit to it.

When Should I Enjoy This Fruit?

I'd advise you to eat your fruit at the end of meals, because fructose, the sugar in the fruit, is a fast sugar. However, if it reaches your digestive tract after the meat and vegetables it will be made to wait with them while a long digestion process takes place, and this slows down the rate at which the sucrose is absorbed as well as its lipogenic (transforming into fat) activity.

Hang on to this principle about physiology: fast sugars aren't allowed to remain in your bloodstream, where they're too dangerous for your eyes, your heart, your brain, your kidneys and the arteries in your lower limbs. Once the sugar in your blood exceeds 10g per litre, it's capable of triggering a diabetic coma if your pancreas doesn't neutralize it by secreting insulin, its ultimate weapon. This hormone, insulin, saves your life. But it also very determinedly expels the sugar from the bloodstream, putting it in quarantine and storing it away as fat.

One portion of fruit contains about 15g sugar, i.e. 3 x 5g sugar cubes. If you lead a sedentary lifestyle, it'll end up on your stomach if you're a man or a menopausal woman, or on your hips and thighs if you're a woman who still has periods.

Also bear in mind that there's a huge difference between whole fruit and fruit juice. Fruit contains soluble fibre in its pulp. Apples, for example, contain pectin, the substance that makes jam set. This fibre really helps to slow down digestion, putting a brake on insulin circulation and weight gain. There is no fibre whatsoever left in fruit juice and so the sugars get into the bloodstream much faster.

Fibre from whole fruit is essential for creating a feeling of satiety. Whichever sort of fruit you choose, it will always be far more filling than its juice. One is eaten, the other is drunk. Furthermore, a glass of fruit juice is almost always the equivalent of at least two pieces of fruit.

Lastly, try and eat your fruit in the evenings if you can. The carbs contained in the fruit may help you to get to sleep and improve the quality of your sleep.

How Should I Enjoy My Fruit?

A further word about fruit.

You must be wondering why I restrict the amount of fruit you're allowed when everywhere you see the recommendation to 'eat five portions of fruit and vegetables a day'. This slogan is ambiguous. What does it mean exactly? Personally, I'd subscribe to it if it meant four vegetables and one fruit, but definitely not the other way round with four fruits and one vegetable. Because there's a clear difference between the two. A vegetable is a fruit but without the sugar. Yes, you read correctly – there's practically no difference in nutritional value and composition between a fruit and a vegetable, the vitamins are strictly the same. A sweet pepper or a cabbage contains just as much vitamin C as the prestigious orange. What sets fruit apart from vegetables is the sugar content. Fruit is full of fructose, for diabetics one of the most dangerous sugars there is, and fattening for anyone trying to control weight problems. Yes, of course, fruit is a natural food, but this doesn't tell us the whole story. Is it natural for man to eat fruit? We have to go right back to the beginnings of the human diet. The fruit we eat nowadays bears no comparison whatsoever with the meagre fruit provided by nature in the wild. The fruit you find in shop displays has been produced using fertilizers and pesticides.

French agronomist Claude Aubert analyzes fruit every year and has shown that it contains 318 different pesticides. He writes in his book *Une autre assiette* (*A different plate,* 2009): 'The skin of the fruit is where most of the antioxidants and vitamins are concentrated. However, it's also where pesticides are concentrated.'

Besides what is an ecological disaster, fruit is one of the foods that make us fat, whereas it's presented to us as a dieting food. One you've attained your True Weight, remember to bear this information in mind.

Oat Bran

The daily amount doesn't change on Wednesday – 1½ tablespoons so you can make your galette.

Konjac

I hope with all my heart that you've got into the habit of eating this fantastic foodstuff. As I've told you, I'm striving to make this easier by improving its availability in any way possible. It always takes a while for new foods to be stocked. I'm also endeavouring to come up with new ready-meal recipes to make life easier for those of you who have no energy left to cook an evening meal after a hectic day.

Wednesday's Drink: Cayenne Pepper and Your Activating Infusion

If you like its spicy taste, carry on making this infusion, which has no contraindications and can do you no harm. A pinch of cayenne pepper a day is a tiny amount, hardly anything – just what you'd use in cooking. The same goes for the green tea, the lime juice and sucralose, which we find everywhere. Try to drink it in two goes, 500ml (18fl oz) with each main meal. Water is an amazing appetite suppressant, green tea helps drain the body and burn a little fat, and the cayenne pepper raises body temperature and acts a little as an appetite suppressant. Drinking it cold at 4°C is an easy way to burn off a few extra calories, too.

Exercise

The further you get into the week, the more you should think about using your body. Apart from the calories burned up through exercising, and the serotonin your brain is made to secrete, physical activity is a fundamental given of animal life. The difference between animal and vegetable is that the latter doesn't move. Vegetable life stays connected to its roots, which soak up goodness from the soil, and to its leaves, where the chlorophyll absorbs the sun's energy. For millions of years, only vegetal species existed. When the animal (animation) kingdom emerged, this was precisely about mobility and movement. No more roots, no more leaves with chlorophyll, but instead now there were bones, muscles, joints, tendons and the instinct to feed and reproduce. For almost a billion years animal life has had to be on the move to ensure its survival.

However, there is more to it than that. If animal life had to be on the move, it had to move efficiently and economically and not be mobile to no good purpose, i.e. it had to move intelligently, using all its brain's resources. And we human beings have the most sophisticated brains of all.

Over the past five years, the international neuroscientific community has made an incredible and radically new discovery. Physical activity, among other things, creates new neurones in the brain from stem cells. This is called **neurogenesis** or, more simply, **brain plasticity**. This discovery has thrown neurological science into disarray. Scarcely ten years ago, we believed that we were born into the world with a fixed supply of neurones and that inevitably we would lose a few thousand each day.

To come back to you, by walking and running, you're burning up calories, you're secreting serotonin and you're maintaining your supply of neurones. So you have everything to gain by being active – you'll lose weight more easily, you'll stoke up your desire to live and you'll remain mentally active for longer.

Your Diet Summary Sheet for Wednesday

Today, on the first Wednesday of your programme, you're allowed Monday's proteins, Tuesday's vegetables and **Wednesday's fruit**.

If you can, try to savour your portion of fruit at the end of your meal, as it's a fast sugar, and preferably in the evening. And, most importantly, stick to the portions you're allowed.

- Lean meats: veal, beef (except rib of beef and rib-eye steak), grilled or roasted without any fat
- Offal: liver, kidneys, and calf's and beef tongue (the tip)

- All fish: oily, lean, white, cooked and uncooked
- All seafood (shellfish and crustaceans)
- All poultry, except goose and duck, and without any skin
- Low-fat, cooked, sliced ham, chicken and turkey
- Eggs
- Vegetable proteins
- Fat-free dairy products
- 1.5 litres (2½ pints) of water (low sodium)
- An oat bran galette or 1½ tablespoons oat bran in milk, yoghurt or fromage frais
- Konjac
- A compulsory 30-minute daily walk
- Your extras: coffee, tea, herbal teas, green tea with cayenne pepper, vinegars, seasonings, herbs, spices, gherkins, lemons, salt and mustard (in moderation)
- All cooked and uncooked vegetables
- One portion of fruit, except bananas, grapes, dried fruit such as dried apricots and prunes, and oleaginous fruits like walnuts, almonds, peanuts, pistachios and other nuts

AND NOTHING ELSE!

DAILY RECIPES

PROTEIN, VEGETABLE AND FRUIT RECIPES FOR **WEDNESDAY**

(and the other days that follow too)

SCALLOPS WITH SPICY ORANGES

(4 servings)
Preparation time: 5 minutes
Cooking time: 10 minutes

24–32 medium-sized scallops (6–8 per serving),
fresh or frozen
2 oranges, peeled and thinly sliced
1 teaspoon ground cinnamon, plus extra for
sprinkling
Grated zest and juice of 2 unwaxed oranges
2 pinches of cayenne pepper
4 tablespoons fat-free fromage frais
4 tablespoons finely chopped fresh coriander
4 pinches of vanilla powder
Salt and black pepper

If you are using frozen scallops, leave them to defrost in some skimmed milk.

Sprinkle the orange slices with some cinnamon.

Warm a non-stick frying pan over a high heat. Add the orange slices and cook for 5 minutes. Remove from the pan and set aside.

Next put the scallops in the pan and stir them gently for 1 minute, just long enough for them to brown slightly.

Add the zest and juice of the 2 unwaxed oranges to the pan along with the cinnamon, cayenne pepper, salt and black pepper, and leave to reduce for about 3 minutes.

Turn the heat right down and add the fromage frais, stirring continuously, and finally the chopped coriander.

Arrange the scallops on top of the cooked orange slices and sprinkle with the vanilla powder.

MINT SORBET WITH STRAWBERRY COULIS

(4 servings)
Preparation time: 10 minutes
Cooking time: 15 minutes

You will need an ice-cream machine

500g (1lb 2oz) strawberries, hulled and halved
1 tablespoon vanilla flavouring

100g (3½oz) virtually fat-free quark
12 tablespoons powdered sweetener
400ml (14fl oz) water
1 bunch of fresh mint

Place the strawberries in a bowl and add the vanilla flavouring, quark and 6 tablespoons of the sweetener. Mix together and then refrigerate.

Bring the water to the boil in a saucepan with the remaining sweetener and the mint (reserve a few mint leaves for decoration). Boil for 15 minutes then leave to infuse until the water has cooled completely.

Sieve the infusion, discarding the mint, and transfer to an ice-cream maker. Churn the sorbet until set.

Serve the mint sorbet with the chilled strawberry coulis poured over the top and decorated with the reserved mint leaves.

SOLE, MANGO AND FENNEL PARCELS

(4 servings)
Preparation time: 15 minutes
Cooking time: 20 minutes

The tart flavour of the mango and fennel combine wonderfully with fromage frais when it melts. A great delicacy, this is an ideal dish for a romantic dinner.

2 fresh mangoes, thinly sliced
1 fennel bulb, thinly sliced
8 fillets of sole
Juice of 2 lemons
A few sprigs of dill
4 tablespoons fat-free fromage frais
100g (3½oz) virtually fat-free quark
Salt and black pepper

Preheat the oven to 180°C/350°F/Gas 4.

To make the parcels, cut out 4 squares of grease-proof paper. Layer each one with mango slices, then fennel and 2 fillets of sole. Finish with a few extra slices of mango on top and then pour over the lemon juice and sprinkle with some dill. Fold up and seal the parcels.

Bake in the oven for 10 minutes. Open up the parcels and divide the fromage frais and quark between them. Season sparingly with salt and black pepper then reseal the parcels and return them to the oven to bake for a further 10 minutes.

VANILLA CHEESECAKE WITH RASPBERRY COULIS

(8 servings)
Preparation time: 25 minutes
Cooking time: 55 minutes + 24 hours chilling

For the biscuit base:
5 tablespoons oat bran
3 tablespoons powdered sweetener, suitable for cooking
150g (5½oz) virtually fat-free quark

For the filling:
375g (13oz) virtually fat-free quark
200g (7oz) fat-free fromage frais
5 tablespoons powdered sweetener, suitable for cooking
3 eggs
1 teaspoon vanilla extract

For the raspberry coulis:
500g (1lb 2oz) raspberries
6 tablespoons powdered sweetener
1 tablespoon lemon juice

First prepare the biscuit base by combining the oat bran with the sweetener and quark. Firmly press the mixture into the bottom and sides of a 17cm (6½in) diameter springform tin with high sides. Refrigerate for 20 minutes.

Preheat the oven to 160°C/325°F/Gas 3.

To make the filling, whisk together the quark, fromage frais and sweetener until you have a really smooth mixture. Next whisk in the eggs, one by one, and then add the vanilla extract.

Pour this mixture over the biscuit base and bake in the preheated oven. After 15 minutes, turn the oven down to 120°C/250°F/Gas ½ and bake for a further 40 minutes. Switch the oven off and leave the cheesecake to cool down inside. Then refrigerate for 24 hours.

In the meantime, prepare the coulis. Press the raspberries through a fine sieve to get rid of the pips. Add the sweetener and lemon juice to the raspberry pulp and refrigerate until ready to serve.

Take the cheesecake out of the fridge, carefully remove it from the tin and serve with the chilled raspberry coulis.

APPLE, PEAR AND RASPBERRY CRUMBLE

(4 servings)
Preparation time: 25 minutes
Cooking time: 25 minutes

Raspberries are not only a delicious fruit, they're very low in sugar. They also aid digestion and are said to help prevent some cancers too, because of the ellagic acid they contain.

Juice of 1 lemon
1 apple, peeled, cored and cubed
2 pears, peeled, cored and cubed
150g (5½oz) raspberries, fresh or frozen
10–15 fresh mint leaves, finely chopped
150g (5½oz) virtually fat-free quark
2 tablespoons oat bran
2 tablespoons powdered sweetener, suitable for cooking

Preheat the oven to 190°C/375°F/Gas 5.

Sprinkle some lemon juice over the apple and pear chunks to prevent them from discolouring. Combine them with the raspberries (defrosted if using frozen) and transfer the fruit to 4 small gratin dishes (or one large ovenproof dish for the family). Sprinkle over the chopped mint.

To make the crumble topping, work the quark into the oat bran and powdered sweetener using your fingers, until the mixture resembles breadcrumbs. Divide the topping between the dishes, without pressing it down. Bake in the oven for 25 minutes.

Allow the crumbles to cool down a little before serving.

EXTRA-LIGHT STRAWBERRY MOUSSE

(4 servings)
Preparation time: 15 minutes + 2 hours chilling
No cooking required

500g (1lb 2oz) strawberries, hulled
1 tablespoon powdered sweetener
A dash of lemon juice
200g (7oz) virtually fat-free quark
3 egg whites

Slice half of the strawberries into quarters and place in a blender. Add the sweetener, lemon juice and quark. Whizz until you get a nice, smooth mixture and transfer to a bowl. Check the sweetness and add more sweetener if necessary.

Cut the remaining strawberries in half and set aside.

Beat the egg whites until they are quite stiff and then gradually fold them into the strawberry mixture using a spatula. Divide the mousse between 4 sundae glasses or ramekin dishes and decorate with the strawberry halves. Chill in the fridge for at least 2 hours before serving.

CITRUS SYLLABUB

(4 servings)
Preparation time: 10 minutes
No cooking required

Very popular in North Africa, orange flower water evokes smells from childhood. You can also use it to make a delicious drink by adding a tablespoon to a cup of hot water with a little sweetener.

1 grapefruit
1 orange
2 mandarins
2 egg yolks
50ml (2fl oz) skimmed milk
2 tablespoons sweetener, suitable for cooking
Orange flower water, to taste

Heat some water in a saucepan large enough to contain a big bowl.

Peel and slice the citrus fruit. Place the fruit in 4 ovenproof dessert ramekin dishes.

In a large, high-sided bowl (which will fit comfortably inside the pan of water) combine the egg yolks, milk, sweetener and orange flower water.

Place the bain-marie bowl in the pan of hot water, and whisk the ingredients for about 5 minutes over a gentle heat until the mixture is nice and frothy.

Pour this mixture over the fruit in the ramekins and warm under a preheated grill for a few seconds before serving.

COCOA ICE CREAM WITH FRESH RASPBERRIES

(4 servings)
Preparation time: 5 minutes
No cooking required

You will need an ice-cream machine

5 tablespoons powdered sweetener
150ml (5fl oz) Dukan Diet 1% fat sugar-free cocoa powder
400ml (14fl oz) boiling water
200g (7oz) virtually fat-free quark

1 teaspoon vanilla extract
4 handfuls of raspberries

In a heatproof bowl, stir together the powdered sweetener and cocoa.

Gradually pour the hot water over the cocoa, whisking the mixture continually until it is nice and smooth. Work in the quark, add the vanilla extract and blend all the ingredients together.

Pour the mixture into an ice-cream maker and churn until set.

When ready to serve, spoon the ice cream into 4 individual bowls and add a handful of raspberries to each.

Thursday

Today, we're climbing up another step on the Nutritional Staircase as we continue to advance.

We started the climb towards your True weight with a Monday devoted exclusively to high-protein foods. Did you know that this is the only vital nutrient? Living without eating any animal proteins KILLS us. And what about vegetarians? you'll say. They get their proteins from cereals, wheat or rice, and from legumes, peas, lentils and beans. However, none of these proteins has all eight of the essential amino acids your body needs to produce its own proteins, in order to keep itself alive.

When you eat animal proteins – for example, meat, fish, eggs, poultry and dairy products – there's a choice of 20 amino acids and among them are these eight essential ones.

As you digest, your body breaks down the long chains made up of smaller amino acid chains, and once they've all been separated, they can enter the bloodstream through the mucous membranes in your intestines.

Once in your blood, they're a bit like Lego or Meccano parts which your body assembles in the only way it knows how – as human proteins, which are different to the animal ones you've eaten. In other words, if you've just eaten a chicken drumstick, you'll have dismantled the chicken structure to reassemble it into a human protein structure.

The proteins in cereals such as wheat, spelt or buck-wheat have one essential amino acid missing, phenylala-nine, and the process gets blocked. You have all the bricks you need, except for one, so you can't build your house.

If you eat legumes, the same thing happens: all the amino acids are there except one. This time it's methio-nine, so once again everything gets blocked.

If you want to produce your vital, human proteins from vegetable ones as vegetarians do, you'll need cereals that are rich in methionine but low in phenylalanine, as well as legumes rich in phenylalanine but lacking methio-nine, and in comparable proportions.

That's not all. Vegetable proteins pose another prob-lem in that they're packed with carbs, i.e. 'sugars'. They may well get slowed down by the fibre in the cereals and legumes, but eating them will impact on weight through mechanisms (i.e. insulin production) which I've described to you often enough.

Up until adolescence proteins are crucial for growth, which cannot happen without them.

Once we reach adulthood they're still vital as we're unable to maintain our bodies and vital organs without them. The body uses these proteins all the time to replace skin, nails and hair, which all form part of our self-image and appearance. The body needs proteins just as much to replenish hormones, muscles, bones, red and white blood cells and even our memory.

What you're reading this very minute will even get recorded in your 'electric' memory, which is the equivalent of your computer's active memory. Over the coming night, thanks to protein molecules, this memory will be stored on your long-term memory's hard drive.

So now you can see why proteins are so vital. The same can't be said for carbs and sugars. Theoretically you could live without them entirely. The Inuits, an Eskimo people who have been studied extensively, live for over seven months a year without any fruit, vegetables or starchy foods. Before American emigrants came on the scene, they survived from eating fish and seals, which meant they had only proteins and fats, no carbs at all and certainly no white sugar or flour. And they were perfectly healthy.

On Tuesday you added vegetables.

Vegetables are not vital foods, but they are essential because they provide vitamins, and we need a minimum intake to survive. Vitamins are found in virtually all food – including proteins.

On Wednesday you were allowed fruit.

Fruit is neither vital nor essential, but it's important nonetheless, as it also provides vitamins along with mineral salts and a few fast sugars, which are useful for people leading an active lifestyle.

I'd like to remind you that, far away from our civilization, Aboriginal peoples ate only 2–3 kilos of sugar a year, whereas the average American today gets through 72 kilos! I believe that this sugar consumption world record explains nutritionally why America has a weight problem epidemic. The societal and behavioural aspect of the problem is that individuals are seeking comfort from sugar to cope with life in the world's main consumer society. And yes, I know, I've said it all before!

Before taking a look at your instruction for Thursday, I'll remind you, as a leitmotif, what the second-front week is based on: Monday to Sunday, each new day brings you a different food group, starting with what's most nutritional and ending with what's most comforting.

Keep this progression in mind. There's great didactic value in repeating it, week after week, until you reach your goal – your True Weight. What you learn from a book, however well explained, speaks to your intellect and can easily be forgotten.

Whereas if you experience something with your own flesh, you are learning through 'being trained' and it gets reinforced through repetition. You're creating a new pathway in your brain as the neurones link up with one another. And once this pathway is well enough established, used and consolidated, it'll become a preferred pathway and hard-wired in your mind forever. Without really noticing it, you'll have acquired good habits and a correct eating pattern. And that's what I'm expecting from you.

Nowadays, hunger and satiety can no longer play the role for us that they play for animals. We're not like the people who lived in the past; they were driven by hunger to do everything they could to feed themselves. Unfortunately, this vital, healthy instinct has all but disappeared. In our present-day brains, our modern, toxic foods create extreme, psychotropic effects. The people who eat because they're hungry are few and far between, and in our consumerist societies there are even fewer who actually stop when they no longer feel hungry. For overweight people and especially for anyone who has tried many different diets, the problem is even greater. These basic physiological sensations have been permanently destroyed. If you recall, I likened this to locks that had been forced. We have to rediscover these sensations. The solution I advocate is to recreate through conditioning an automatic-pilot tool, so that you control your eating within a structured system. Trust me, everything can be learnt; or in your case, to be more precise, can be re-learnt.

This is one of the roles of the Nutritional Staircase.

Today, Thursday, we've reached the limit of the week's weight-loss section. Although at the end of the race, we've still got some of our initial momentum left. Sailors talk about 'headway' to describe the speed a boat can maintain once the engine has been more or less switched off.

As you'll be anticipating, today we're going to add another food and this time it's **bread.** If you're still with me, you can make a shrewd guess that we're not talking about white bread here, but brown bread, wholemeal bread and, if at all possible, wholegrain bread.

White bread means white flour. White flour is ground to be as fine as possible, refined and purified. Industry does all this work so there's nothing left for your body to do. This means that the flour or white bread travels through your digestive tract, from your mouth to your small intestine, at lightning speed, and at the same speed as your blood glucose. No doubt you're beginning to work out what will happen next – weight gain caused by insulin secretion and sugar turned into fat.

So what I'm offering you today is wholegrain or wholemeal bread. What's the difference between them?

Wholegrain bread is made from whole wheat, by which I mean that it's harvested then ground without separating the fibrous husk or bran from the wheat. The glycaemic index for wholegrain bread is lower (40) than for wholemeal bread (50) because it hasn't undergone any sifting. The flour used to make it contains all the wheat seed components: the wheat kernel's husk and germ (fibre, essential fatty acids, vitamins and mineral salts).

Wholemeal bread is made with white flour to which wheat is added – it's a reconstituted food. And it's completely different. The bran and its husk make up a unit whose parts are naturally welded together. Once they've been separated by industrial processes, the flour and bran can be put back together, but now they're only attached and no longer welded by their natural links. As soon as you put this bread in your mouth and it reaches the stomach in lightning speed, the white flour's sugars immediately separate from the wheat bran's slow sugars. So watch out!

Therefore the instruction for Thursday is clear: **you keep all Monday's high-protein foods, still eating as much as you want, the same goes for Tuesday's vegetables and you keep Wednesday's fruit too.**

AND TODAY, YOU'RE ALLOWED TWO SLICES OF WHOLEGRAIN BREAD

Two slices is equivalent to 45g (1oz).
Be careful: if you have your bread for breakfast you aren't allowed any butter or jam. However, you can eat it with some cooked turkey, fat-free cream cheese or cottage cheese, a nice slice of smoked salmon; or you can have it alongside a boiled egg, fried egg or scrambled egg. Personally, I'd suggest you keep your oat bran galette for the mornings and enjoy your bread at some other time of the day.

If you have your bread at lunchtime, you can combine it with whatever you're allowed, meat or fish. Better still, you can use it to make a sandwich and add some ham, lettuce and a few slices of tomato. Why not try some bresaola or chicken liver spread.

If you'd rather keep your two slices for the evening, take a little time to make some French toast, a pissaladière tart or some other treat. You could also turn the bread into crumbs to add texture to your main dishes.

Oat Bran

On Thursdays you stick to your 1½ tablespoons of oat bran. If you'd rather have your bread than an oat bran galette for breakfast, then keep the oat bran to make something else. There are all sorts of sweet (using sweetener, of course) and savoury recipes – you could make traditional muffins or blinis, or even a pizza base perfect for the topping of your choice: tomatoes, anchovies, fromage frais mixed with quark or cream cheese, herbs, a few peeled prawns or strips of smoked salmon. The possibilities are vast, so be adventurous and let yourself be guided by what you most enjoy.

Konjac

No change here, the instruction remains the same – you're allowed total freedom and variety in your dishes. Learn how best to use konjac as it offers you a fantastic way to lose weight easily. Experiment with ways of cooking it so that konjac becomes part of your repertoire – as I keep telling you, it has no calories. You stand the best chance of keeping the weight off if you eat konjac.

Thursday's Drink: Green Tea and Cayenne Pepper Infusion

Carry on drinking your litre (1¾ pints) of green tea, with its pinch of cayenne pepper, lime juice and sucralose. Always drink it nice and cold and get your body to produce thermogenesis to offset the coldness of the drink and burn up a few more calories.

If you don't like this infusion, then drink 1.5 litres (2½ pints) of water.

Exercise

The further you get through the week, the more important it becomes to keep to your half an hour of walking, jogging, swimming or dancing. Don't give up on this route to vitality, energy and physical fitness because sooner or later you'll feel the benefits. If you persevere, you'll make the connection between what may perhaps seem to you to be superfluous effort and the well-being it'll bring you. Try it and you'll see it's true – just think about what I've told you regarding serotonin.

Whatever your age, this neurotransmitter must be and must remain a key element in your life. Realizing this, and I mean truly realizing it through having experimented with it and experienced it personally, is the most valuable guide. It helps you to see life differently. The day you become fully aware of this fact, as happened with me, you'll be able to adjust your priorities in life, and believe you me, that's no small achievement.

We are each born with our own particular temperament, family history and initial programming. During the first few months of their lives, babies develop in an environment of immediate survival, until they reach their first developmental threshold, the 'imprint' threshold. Next they pass into the hands of those who mould and shape them by instilling the prevailing culture until they reach the second threshold of maturity at the end of adolescence. And from then on our supreme, but subconscious, goal in life is to get enough serotonin, which is achieved through behaviour patterns that are driven by our nature and acceptable to our culture. If a person's life journey, family, environment and opportunities have been favourable, he or she will have a certain number of ways of accessing this 'food', the most precious of all physical and symbolic foods, as it's the sustenance that makes us enjoy life so that we try to stay alive each new day.

Your Diet Summary Sheet for Thursday

Today, on the first Thursday of your programme, added to Monday's proteins, Tuesday's vegetables and Wednesday's fruit are **Thursday's two slices of wholegrain or wholemeal bread.**

As I've explained, try and stick to wholegrain, or failing that wholemeal bread, but definitely avoid all white bread as it's made with white flour.

On Thursday, you finish your weight-loss phase and move into a stabilization phase on Friday.

Thursday

- Lean meats: veal, beef (except rib of beef and rib-eye steak), grilled or roasted without any fat
- Offal: liver, kidneys, and calf's and beef tongue (the tip)
- All fish: oily, lean, white, cooked and uncooked
- All seafood (shellfish and crustaceans)
- All poultry, except goose and duck, and without any skin
- Low-fat, cooked, sliced ham, chicken and turkey
- Eggs
- Vegetable proteins
- Fat-free dairy products
- 1.5 litres (2½ pints) of water (low sodium)
- An oat bran galette or 1½ tablespoons oat bran in milk, yoghurt or fromage frais
- Konjac
- A compulsory 30-minute daily walk
- Your extras: coffee, tea, herbal teas, green tea with cayenne pepper, vinegars, seasonings, herbs, spices, gherkins, lemons, salt and mustard (in moderation)
- All cooked and uncooked vegetables
- One portion of fruit, except bananas, grapes, dried fruit such as dried apricots and prunes, and oleaginous fruits like walnuts, almonds, peanuts, pistachios and other nuts
- Two slices of wholegrain or wholemeal bread

AND NOTHING ELSE!

DAILY RECIPES

PROTEIN, VEGETABLE, FRUIT AND BREAD RECIPES FOR **THURSDAY**

(and the other days that follow too)

HERB SALAD QUARTET WITH SAINT-PIERRELIN ON TOAST

(4 servings)
Preparation time: 10 minutes
Cooking time: 5 minutes

4 different lettuces (e.g. butterhead, curly endive, lollo rosso, escarole), weighing a total of 300g (10½oz)
6 tablespoons Maya Salad Dressing (see page 156)
½ teaspoon Dukan Diet honey flavouring
1 shallot, finely chopped
1 onion, finely chopped
4 tablespoons quark
8 small slices of wholemeal bread
To serve:
A few chopped basil leaves
A few chopped chives
A few chopped tarragon leaves

Thursday

Rinse the lettuce leaves and divide between 4 serving plates.

In a bowl, mix together the dressing, honey flavouring, shallot and onion.

Mix the quark in the bowl with salt and the oregano. Spread it on slices of toast.

Arrange 2 slices of toast on each plate and divide the dressing between them. Sprinkle over the chopped chives, basil and tarragon to serve.

PISSALADIÈRE SLICES

(4 servings)
Preparation time: 30 minutes
Cooking time: 25 minutes

600g (1lb 5oz) sweet onions, thinly sliced
1 teaspoon herbes de Provence, plus extra to garnish
1 tablespoon mustard
4 large slices of wholemeal or Poilâne bread
12 anchovy fillets, oil-free or wiped
Salt and black pepper

Add 3 drops of oil to a frying pan then wipe off with kitchen paper and fry the onions. Season with salt

213

and black pepper and cook for about 30 minutes, adding a little water if necessary and stirring at regular intervals, until the onions have browned very slightly. Mix in the herbes de Provence and set aside.

Preheat the oven to 180°C/350°F/Gas 4.

Spread the mustard over the slices of bread, then add a layer of onions and top with the anchovy fillets.

Sprinkle over a few extra herbes de Provence and bake in the oven for 25 minutes.

TUNA PROVENÇAL SLICES

(4 servings)
Preparation time: 10 minutes
No cooking required

I prefer the subtler taste of white albacore tuna to that of red tuna. With this recipe, you can replace the cucumber, pepper and fennel with thinly sliced pink radish.

1 tin tuna in brine
200g (7oz) virtually fat-free quark
A dash of lemon juice
Freshly ground white pepper

2 tablespoons finely chopped basil
4 large slices of wholemeal or Poilâne bread
1 cucumber, sliced
1 red pepper, cut into thin strips
1 fennel bulb, cut into thin strips

Drain the tuna and flake it into a blender. Add the quark along with the lemon juice and white pepper. Blend until you have a nice smooth mixture, then stir in the basil.

Toast the bread. Mix the cucumber, pepper and fennel into the tuna mixture and spread over the toasted bread slices. Arrange the slices on a serving dish and enjoy either as an appetizer with drinks or a tasty starter.

ORANGE AND RED STRIPED SALMON SLICES

(4 servings)
Preparation time: 10 minutes + 2 hours chilling
Cooking time: 15 minutes

300g (10½oz) fresh salmon
2 small fennel bulbs, thinly sliced
2 tablespoons balsamic vinegar
Juice of 2 lemons
Dukan Mayonnaise (see below)

A few chives, finely chopped
4 large slices of wholemeal or Poilâne bread
Salt and black pepper

Cut half of the salmon into small cubes and mix together with the fennel, balsamic vinegar, half of the lemon juice, some salt and black pepper. Stir well and refrigerate for at least 2 hours.

Meanwhile, preheat the oven to 160°C/325°F/Gas 3, and cook the rest of the salmon for 15 minutes.

Once the salmon has cooled down, flake it and add some Dukan mayonnaise, half the remaining lemon juice and some chopped chives. Season and refrigerate for at least 1 hour.

Lightly toast the bread and spread some of the cooked salmon down one edge. Then spread some of the fennel and salmon mixture alongside. Repeat the alternating stripes of salmon mixture to cover the toast slices and refrigerate until you are ready to serve, drizzled with the remaining lemon juice.

Dukan Mayonnaise: mix an egg yolk with a tablespoon of Dijon mustard, 3 tablespoons of virtually fat-free fromage frais or quark and some salt and black pepper. This makes enough for 2 portions. Must be kept chilled.

CROSTINI SLICES WITH MELON AND BRESAOLA

(4 servings)
Preparation time: 20 minutes
Cooking time: 5 minutes

½ melon, halved and deseeded
100g (3½oz) bresaola
2 tablespoons balsamic vinegar
1 teaspoon Dukan Diet honey flavouring
4 large slices of wholemeal or Poilâne bread
1 garlic clove
⅓ bunch of basil, finely chopped
Fleur de sel or sea salt flakes and black pepper

Remove the skin from the melon and chop the flesh into small cubes. Cut the bresaola lengthways into strips. Combine the melon with the bresaola and season with 1 tablespoon of the balsamic vinegar and the honey flavouring. Leave to rest in the fridge.

Preheat the grill. Rub the slices of bread with the garlic clove and brush the remaining vinegar over them. Toast under the grill for a few minutes.

Remove the melon mixture from the fridge and season with some sea salt and a little freshly ground black pepper. Add the chopped basil.

Spread the melon tartare over each of the bread slices and serve.

MEDITERRANEAN SLICES

(4 servings)
Preparation time: 15 minutes
Cooking time: 1 minute

Feta is a Greek speciality, a curd cheese made from goat's or ewe's milk.

4 large slices of wholemeal or Poilâne bread
4 lettuce leaves, chopped
8 cherry tomatoes, halved
160g (5¾oz) feta cheese, cubed
4 sundried tomatoes, cut into petals
½ red pepper, sliced
1 hard-boiled egg, quartered
16 basil leaves
A few thin slices of red onion
2 tablespoons Maya Salad Dressing (see page 156)

Lightly toast the bread and arrange the lettuce on top.

Place the cherry tomatoes and feta on top of the lettuce, followed by the sundried tomatoes and red pepper.

Place an egg quarter on each slice then scatter over a few basil leaves and onion slices.

To serve, dribble ½ tablespoon of the dressing over each slice of toast.

SARDINIAN BRUSCHETTA

(4 servings)
Preparation time: 20 minutes + 2 hours marinating
Cooking time: 5 minutes

8 tinned sardine fillets, in brine or oil
Juice of 2 limes
1 preserved lemon
2 large tomatoes
4 large slices of wholegrain bread
1 garlic clove
150g (5½oz) virtually fat-free quark
100g (3½oz) anchovies in brine
8 sundried tomatoes, cut into petals
1 small onion, finely chopped
1 small fennel bulb, finely chopped
2 tablespoons capers
Thyme and rosemary
Fleur de sel or sea salt flakes and freshly ground black pepper

If you are using sardine fillets in oil, carefully wipe off all the oil with some kitchen paper. Place the fillets in a dish and pour over the lime juice. Cut the preserved lemon into small pieces and scatter over the sardines. Cover the dish with cling film and leave to marinate for 2 hours.

Peel and dice the tomatoes, and season with sea salt and black pepper.

Preheat the oven to 200°C/400°F/Gas 6.

Place the bread on a baking tray and bake in the oven for 5 minutes. Remove from the oven and rub the bread with a garlic clove.

Mash the quark with the anchovy fillets and spread the mixture over the bread slices. Then add the diced tomatoes, dried tomato petals, onion, fennel and capers. Season with thyme and rosemary.

Finally add the marinated sardines and serve immediately.

Friday

We continue our climb as today we come to the fifth step of the Nutritional Staircase.

Having followed it from the beginning, you now know that, as we move upwards, **we automatically keep whatever was gained the previous day and add to it what we gain today.**

So this means that added to Monday's high-protein food base are Tuesday's vegetables, Wednesday's fruit and Thursday's two slices of wholegrain or wholemeal bread.

Up to this point, we've been continually on the move, with your metabolism in a combustion phase that meant you were burning off part of your fat reserves, a small part but a part nonetheless.

AND TODAY I'M ADDING A PORTION OF CHEESE

Imagine a pair of scales. On the one side are the foods to which we keep adding day after day, and on the other side is your body, which is having to dip into its reserves as it can't make do with what you're feeding it. With yesterday's two slices of bread it was just about able to reach a point of neutrality, but energy expenditure remained slightly above intake, so it still had to draw on its reserves.

However, with this portion of cheese that I'm now placing on the fifth step of your Nutritional Staircase, I'm bringing you to a point of equilibrium where the two sides of the scales are at the same level. Nutritionally speaking, we say that energy intake matches energy expenditure. A traditional 'balanced diet' is comprised of the food that Friday offers.

At the same time, this demonstrates very concretely that if you want to lose weight, this idea of a balanced diet is not the answer. Why is this so?

BY DEFINITION, PUTTING ON WEIGHT
IS THE RESULT OF AN IMBALANCE

To have put on weight, you must have eaten too many carbs and fats. In other words, you've eaten an unbalanced diet, too high in white bread, pasta, potatoes, refined cereals and rice, and starchy foods; or, worse, too high in white sugar, brown sugar or any colour of sugar, and fizzy drinks; and no doubt you've snacked your way through a range of biscuits, chocolate bars and spreads. And let's not forget the excesses of all those high-fat foods: oil, butter, cream, chocolate, cheese and cooked deli meats. There's no point trying to deny it, eating 'a little too much' of these foods always results in weight gain. With such excesses, a double imbalance creeps into your diet – quantitative (calories from the fats) and qualitative (insulin production from the sugars).

For a person with a normal weight and metabolism, this double imbalance will make them put on weight. So it's easy for you to see how a simple balanced diet, such as the one you're trying this morning, doesn't have any hope of making you lose weight if you're already overweight. This sort of diet can only keep your weight in balance and prevent you from putting on more, BUT it isn't going to make you lose any weight whatsoever. Healthy, balanced diets such as the Mediterranean diet, the Cretan diet and the Okinawa diet are astonishingly good for maintaining a steady weight but they don't work as weight-loss diets.

BUT YOU DO WANT TO LOSE WEIGHT!

You want to get rid of a few unwanted pounds or a stone or so. To actually lose weight, you'll have to follow a low-fat, low-sugar diet. So, in a certain way, if logic and common sense prevail, this could be called an 'unbalanced' diet! I've often been criticized for this, which is quite ironic, isn't it? Since with today's global weight problem epidemic, it's really our current diet that's the *unbalanced* one. Even if we eat less than people did in the past, we consume far too much fat and aggressive sugar and not nearly enough vegetables or proteins. To help you lose weight, my diet tackles, point by point, what makes you fat. As simple as this may sound, during the weight-loss period it replaces an imbalance in sugars and fats with an imbalance of vegetables and proteins, i.e. my 100 'as much as you want' foods.

Let me tell you a little about fats.

The debate about fats has been raging among medics for some time now, as people have tried to determine which of the two nutrients – carbs or fats – is most responsible for creating weight problems and obesity. Many medical historians and sociologists have endeavoured to decipher the reasons that led first the United States, and then the rest of the world, to be battling as we are against cholesterol, and to understand the repercussions of this on our health and the economy.

Around the mid-1960s, weight problems were not the huge problem in America they've since become. Just like anywhere else in the world, the popular way of losing weight was to cut out bread, pasta, potatoes and cakes, which amounted to pointing the finger of blame at carbs.

Then there came a bombshell. Following a few studies that highlighted the relationship between hypercholesterolemia and cardiovascular mortality, cholesterol and animal fat were singled out as responsible for the heart attacks occurring with ever greater frequency among our friends on the other side of the Atlantic. This hypothesis, which should have been confirmed by the medical profession, was seized upon straightaway by the media, inflaming public opinion. Very soon the matter was whipped up to become a public safety issue, the Americans are good at this – cholesterol was demonized and systematically tracked down, to the extent that blood tests were carried out in supermarkets, which shows just how far things went. At the same time the voices of those who were asking for time to assess and reflect, worried that the wrong adversary had been identified, went unheard. The cholesterol hunt was then extended to include all fats. And here I'd like to draw your attention to a decisive moment in the history of weight problems, obesity and diabetes: banishing fats almost automatically cleared sugar of all wrongdoing. Basically, what the people in charge of nutrition said was, 'Eat as little fat as possible but as much sugar as you want,' which left the way wide open for the sugar and flour industries. At the same time calorie-counting was advocated and the daily amount of carbs in a Western diet for people leading a sedentary lifestyle was laid down as having to be strictly 55–60 per cent.

However, American national statistics showed that despite this war against fats, the number of heart attacks did not drop over the following decade. Quite the reverse, in fact – this was the time when the obesity and diabetes epidemic exploded.

Forty years on, statins (anti-cholesterol drugs) remain one of the most widely sold types of medication across the globe. Millions of people use them and will be required to take them for the rest of their lives. If you're overweight, you're likely to be dealing with cholesterol and therefore will be on statins.

And so the debate continues ... Prestigious doctors with quite opposing views are continually at loggerheads. Some think statins are necessary, although they come with potentially terrible side effects, such as extremely painful muscular problems and hepatotoxicity. For others, such as French specialists Professors Debré and Phillipe Even, cholesterol plays no significant part in cardiovascular disease and in any case contributes far less than stress, lifestyle and being physically inactive. The most committed advocate of this viewpoint, Doctor Michel de Lorgeril from the French National Centre for Scientific Research (CNRS), states that 'we're unavoidably driven to the conclusion that these medicines are useless and dangerous and should be withdrawn from the market'.

I've told you this story because it lies at the heart of my commitment to fighting weight problems. When I look back on the fact that weight problems are a major collateral damage resulting from our 'economic growth', which has no scruples as regards public health, I am comforted to see that the director general of WHO recognized and denounced this in a recent speech (see 'Fighting at your side', pages 384–6), unambiguously laying the blame for our obesity pandemic at the door of manufacturers who produce processed sugary and starchy foods.

Coming back to your cheese, it does of course contain fat. But remember that the Cretans, who are the biggest cheese eaters in the world, also have the lowest incidence of heart attacks!

So I've added one portion of cheese to the Nutritional Staircase and you're allowed 40g (1½oz), a proper day's portion, for whichever meal you wish and you can divide it out over the day, too.

What Cheese Am I Allowed?

Any cheese is allowed that doesn't contain more than 45–50% fat.
This means you're allowed hard rind cheeses such as Gouda, Edam, Tomme de Savoie, Mimolette, Comté or reduced fat cheddar, and soft rind cheeses such as Camembert, goat's cheese, Cantal and Reblochon.

Can I share a little secret with you? I always opt for Tomme de Savoie, which in France comes in many versions ranging from 12% to 40% fat. I prefer the 12% fat version myself – try it, it's surprisingly good. It's made with semi-skimmed milk to the same recipe that was used up until the Second World War. Then, to suit the post-war generation, the fat content was increased. Nowadays, with people watching their weight, manufacturers have gone back to their original recipe and even sell a 10% fat version.

Remember, too, that Parmesan with its strong taste

contains only 30% fat, and is great, for example, for adding flavour to your konjac shiratakis.

Friday is a neutral day, when the week is in suspension, when you don't lose weight or gain it.

This is a welcome balance, except for those who have difficulty losing weight, the most obvious case being anyone suffering from an underactive thyroid as a deficiency in the thyroid hormone slows down metabolism. People who take cortisones and many anti-depressants may also find that they gain some weight because of these medicines. Anyone who is really inactive and refuses to take any exercise is likely to put on a little as well. Conversely, some people who are usually described as 'easy cases' may find that they even lose a little weight.

Oat Bran

The instruction remains the same, keep to the same dose, $1\frac{1}{2}$ tablespoons, just what you need to make your oat bran galette.

Remember again that not all brans are the same. So check that the one you're using isn't too fine. Ideally it should be milled to produce medium-sized particles and sifted sufficiently so that it doesn't contain any naturally sweet oat flour. Try blowing gently on the bran to see if this lifts off any flour.

Konjac

The same prescription here, too. Eat as much as you want; the more you eat, the more weight you'll lose. Like oat bran, konjac is very filling. Oat bran is a cereal (pasta) equivalent and konjac a starchy food (rice) equivalent.

Friday's Drink: Green Tea and Cayenne Pepper Infusion

Keep to the following ingredients for your infusion: 15g (½oz) green tea leaves or green tea pearls for 1 litre (1¾ pints) of water, a pinch of cayenne pepper, the juice of ½ lime and 3 teaspoons of sucralose. Drink it nice and cold to burn a few calories with no extra effort.

Once again, remember that water is the best natural, automatic appetite suppressant.

Tomorrow, as it's the weekend, we'll adapt the recipe so that the infusion offers you added protection.

Exercise

I've spoken enough about this on previous days. Keep to your 30-minute walk today and try to listen to what is going on inside you. Perhaps you'll start to hear a noise coming from your serotonin source.

Your Diet Summary Sheet for Friday

Today, on the first Friday of your programme, as well as Monday's proteins, Tuesday's vegetables, Wednesday's fruit and Thursday's two slices of bread, you're allowed **one portion of cheese**.

Friday is the neutral day of the week, a day when you're in suspension, neither losing nor gaining weight.

- Lean meats: veal, beef (except rib of beef and rib-eye steak), grilled or roasted without any fat
- Offal: liver, kidneys, and calf's and beef tongue (the tip)
- All fish: oily, lean, white, cooked and uncooked
- All seafood (shellfish and crustaceans)
- All poultry, except goose and duck, and without any skin
- Low-fat, cooked, sliced ham, chicken and turkey
- Eggs
- Vegetable proteins
- Fat-free dairy products
- 1.5 litres (2½ pints) of water (low sodium)
- An oat bran galette or 1½ tablespoons oat bran in milk, yoghurt or fromage frais
- Konjac
- A compulsory 30-minute daily walk
- Your extras: coffee, tea, herbal teas, green tea with cayenne pepper, vinegars, seasonings, herbs, spices, gherkins, lemons, salt and mustard (in moderation)
- All cooked and uncooked vegetables
- One portion of fruit, except bananas, grapes, dried fruit such as dried apricots and prunes, and oleaginous fruits like walnuts, almonds, peanuts, pistachios and other nuts
- Two slices of wholegrain or wholemeal bread
- One portion of hard or soft rind cheese, less than 50% fat

AND NOTHING ELSE!

DAILY RECIPES

PROTEIN, VEGETABLE, FRUIT, BREAD AND CHEESE RECIPES FOR **FRIDAY**

(and for the other days that follow)

SMALL SQUASH WITH COMTÉ

(4 servings)
Preparation time: 10 minutes
Cooking time: 20 minutes

Nutmeg used to be well known for calming respiratory difficulties. But did you know that it's also found in the (top secret) list of ingredients for Coca-Cola?

4 onion (red kuri) squashes, or similar
160g (5¾oz) Comté cheese, sliced
4 pinches of grated nutmeg
Salt and black pepper

Preheat the oven to 180°C/350°F/Gas 4.

Cut the 'lid' off the top of each squash and remove the seeds. Rinse the insides.

Fill the cavities with the cheese, season with salt and black pepper and finish off with a pinch of nutmeg. Bake in the oven for 20 minutes.

Serve piping hot.

BEEF CARPACCIO WITH PARMESAN

(4 servings)
Preparation time: 15 minutes + 30 minutes chilling
No cooking required

Juice of 3 lemons
8 slices of rump steak, very thinly sliced
250g (9oz) button mushrooms, thinly sliced
160g (5¾oz) Parmesan cheese, shaved
A few fresh basil leaves, finely chopped
A few rocket leaves
8 small slices of wholegrain bread
Salt and black pepper

Mix the lemon juice with some salt and black pepper.

Arrange the steak on 4 plates, spreading out the slices. Pour over the lemon juice and place the mushrooms on top with the Parmesan shavings and basil. Cover the plates with cling film and leave in the fridge for 30 minutes, until you are ready to serve.

Arrange some rocket leaves in the centre of each plate and serve with the slices of wholegrain bread.

MUSHROOM, BRESAOLA AND FRUITY GOUDA SLICES

(4 servings)
Preparation time: 10 minutes
Cooking time: 10 minutes

If you enjoy stronger flavours, replace the fruity Gouda with mature Gouda.

4 large slices of Poilâne bread (or 8 small slices of wholegrain bread)
8 slices of bresaola, cut into thin strips
2 shallots, finely chopped
250g (9oz) button mushrooms, thinly sliced
Juice of 1 lemon
160g (5¾oz) fruity Gouda cheese, grated
Salt and black pepper

Preheat the oven to 200°C /400°F/Gas 6.

Place the slices of bread on a baking sheet and bake in the oven for 2 minutes.

In the meantime, place the bresaola strips in a non-stick frying pan, add the shallots and fry for 3 minutes. Add the mushrooms, turn up the heat and cook for a further 5 minutes. Season with salt and black pepper.

Deglaze using the lemon juice. If necessary, adjust the seasoning and then divide the mixture between the slices of bread. Sprinkle over the grated cheese then put the bread slices back in the oven for about 10 minutes. Finish off under the grill if the Gouda hasn't fully melted.

MOUNTAIN SALAD WITH TOMME DE SAVOIE

(4 servings)
Preparation time: 20 minutes
No cooking required

For the salad:
4 green apples, peeled and quartered
Juice of 1 lemon
1 lettuce, leaves separated
2 chicory heads, leaves separated
160g (5¾oz) Tomme de Savoie cheese, thinly sliced
Fresh parsley, finely chopped
For the dressing:
8–10 tablespoons Maya Salad Dressing (see page 156)
2 tablespoons walnut vinegar
½ teaspoon Dukan Diet walnut flavouring (optional)
Salt and black pepper

Sprinkle the apples with the lemon juice.

Make the dressing by mixing together all the ingredients. You can use both walnut vinegar and walnut flavouring, if you like, for a richer dressing.

Arrange the lettuce and chicory leaves on 4 plates, and spread the apples and cheese on top. Pour the dressing over the salad and garnish with the chopped parsley.

CARPACCIO OF FRESH SALMON AND GOAT'S CHEESE

(4 servings)
Preparation time: 10 minutes + 30 minutes marinating
No cooking required

If you're not fond of goat's cheese, replace it with very thin slices of mozzarella.

200g (7oz) fresh salmon, very thinly sliced
Juice of 2 lemons
1 shallot, finely chopped
1 tablespoon finely chopped dill
1 fresh goat's cheese log
8 small slices of wholegrain bread
Rocket leaves
Fleur de sel or sea salt flakes and black pepper

Line 4 plates with the salmon slices.

Mix together the lemon juice, shallot and dill and use a brush to coat the salmon in this marinade.

Cut the goat's cheese log into 8–12 small slices. Place 2–3 slices on each plate and drizzle over some of the marinade.

Season with a little salt and black pepper and cover with cling film before refrigerating for 30 minutes.

Meanwhile, toast the wholegrain bread. Serve the salmon carpaccio with the toasted bread and some rocket leaves.

SPINACH AND GOAT'S CHEESE GRATIN

(4 servings)
Preparation time: 15 minutes
Cooking time: 20 minutes

400g (14oz) frozen spinach
2 tablespoons fat-free fromage frais
160g (5¾oz) log-style goat's cheese, thinly sliced
250ml (9fl oz) skimmed milk
2 eggs
Grated nutmeg
Salt and black pepper

Preheat the oven to 180°C/350°F/Gas 4.

In a saucepan, thaw and cook the spinach over a gentle heat for 10 minutes and then drain thoroughly. Stir the fromage frais into the spinach.

Lightly oil a gratin dish using some kitchen paper. Build up alternate layers of cheese and spinach.

In a large bowl, whisk together the skimmed milk, eggs and nutmeg and season with salt and black pepper. Pour into the gratin dish and bake in the oven for 20 minutes.

CHICORY AND MATURE MIMOLETTE SALAD

(4 servings)
Preparation time: 10 minutes
No cooking required

This recipe also works really well if you replace the chicory with diced artichoke hearts. The artichoke and Mimolette combination is rather unusual, but very tasty. Serve with wholemeal bread or an oat bran galette.

400g (14oz) fat-free cottage cheese
160g (5¾oz) mature or extra-mature Mimolette (or mature cheddar)

cheese, shaved
4 chicory heads, leaves separated
A few chives, finely chopped
1 teaspoon 5 peppercorn mix
4 tablespoons Maya Salad Dressing (see page 156)
Sherry vinegar

Put some cottage cheese in the centre of each plate with the Mimolette shavings, and arrange the chicory leaves all around like flower petals. Sprinkle the chopped chives over the cottage cheese, and the 5 peppercorn mix over everything. Then pour one tablespoon of dressing over the chicory leaves along with a dash of sherry vinegar.

Saturday

THE LEITMOTIF
Monday for what's vital
Tuesday for what's essential
Wednesday for what's important
Thursday for what's useful
Friday for what's smooth and creamy
Saturday for energy
and Sunday for freedom!

Today we're placing our foot on the last but one step of our Nutritional Staircase and the weekend starts with Saturday. We're close to the top now, which means we've moved into the reward and relaxation zone. This is where you've been heading since Tuesday when vegetables were added, followed by fruit, bread and cheese, and is the step before you reach the culmination, scheduled for tomorrow – Sunday.

I described yesterday, Friday, as a neutral day when both sides of the eating scales were in balance (energy intake equalling energy expenditure).

Today I'm pleased to tell you that I'm adding a pure carbohydrate food. You know what I think about introducing carbs into a diet where we're trying to achieve weight loss. So, let me warn you now that this latest addition will leave the way open for a slight weight gain. **Don't worry – my overall system is designed in such a way that any weight gain this weekend will not in any way endanger what you've achieved so far and it will be far less than the weight you've lost during the first four days**. However, for this to happen, we'll need to take a few precautions.

AND TODAY I'M ADDING A PORTION OF STARCHY FOODS

In addition to the proteins, vegetables, fruit, two slices of bread and portion of cheese, you're allowed one portion of starchy foods today.

I'm going to be very specific now so that there's no room for any mistakes or misunderstandings.

- Firstly, you must weigh out this portion, at least the first time, and you have to weigh your starchy foods cooked and not uncooked. Pasta, for example, doubles in weight as it absorbs the water it's cooked in.
- Secondly, this portion varies in amount according to the type of starchy food you choose.

Starchy foods, as the name suggests, are starch-based. It's a rather hotch-potch food group. Potatoes, cereals and legumes all get grouped together under the term 'starchy foods'.

Among cereals we find wheat, rye, rice, spelt, barley, oats, corn, quinoa and all their by-products – bulgur, groats, polenta and pasta. And then for legumes, you've got peas, lentils and the huge bean family.

If you want to stabilize the weight loss you've achieved, you need to understand that all carbohydrate-containing foods, whatever they are – bread, flour, pasta, rice, potatoes etc. – are made up of a foundation brick, an ultra-fast sugar, which, once it's been taken apart and assimilated, enters the bloodstream as glucose. Whether you have a sugar cube, a spoonful of honey or a tablespoonful of lentils or quinoa, once they've been stripped and dismantled, all these carbohydrate-containing foods release a certain amount of glucose.

However, there is a difference between these various types of carbohydrate-containing foods – plants and starchy foods are made up of different internal textures. To extract the sugar contained within them, your body has first to break down the barriers in the cell wall structure that encloses and contains the sugar. The more resistant this structure is, the longer it takes for the work to be done and for the sugar to be extracted, digested and assimilated.

Whenever these fibrous cell walls are few and far between and disintegrate quickly, we talk about fast sugars. We talk of slow sugars if there is enough of a cell wall structure and enough resistance to slow down their release. However, nowadays you'll hear people use the term 'invasive power' when referring to quickly absorbed carbs, and 'gradual power' for carbs that are absorbed slowly, with less emphasis on the notion of speed.

Remember that the greater or quicker this absorption of sugar is, the more toxic the concentration of glucose in the bloodstream will be for your vital organs – heart, eyes, kidneys, arteries and brain.

This toxic absorption has to be immediately neutralized by an appropriate dose of insulin. Insulin knows only one way to protect your life and that is to dispatch this sugar to the single part of your body that is willing to accept so much so quickly, i.e. the fat tissues.

Starchy foods are one of the high-carb foods that have enough fibrous plant texture to slow down sugar absorption and allow the body's cells to use the carbs as fuel because they are gradually absorbed and then assimilated. Thanks to this fibrous texture, less insulin is secreted and so less fat is produced, and consequently the potential risk of diabetes decreases as well.

However useful this particular feature of starchy foods might be, it must not make us forget that they still contain sugar, which all too often is what tends to happen. Admittedly, the blood glucose level rises gradually and is less brutal, but if you eat a significant quantity of starchy foods this may produce concentrations as high as if you'd been eating cakes and pastries.

We're led to believe nowadays that fast sugars are

radically different from slow sugars and that sweets are totally unlike potatoes, but we're mistaken here. After a plateful of pasta or mashed potato our blood sugar level may rise a little more slowly but it will still rise to almost the same extent. This means that a diabetic, pre-diabetic or obese person, who believes in this oversimplified contrast between fast and slow sugars and makes a beeline for starchy foods in the belief that it's the healthy option, would be quite mistaken and would be doing so to their own detriment.

To be sure, a meal with pasta or white rice may be less aggressive for the body than eating honey, white flour or mashed potato, but harmless it certainly isn't.

As far as starchy foods are concerned, I'd personally advise eating them in moderation for normal weight and non-diabetic inactive people, with care if you're overweight, and if you're obese or diabetic you should avoid them altogether.

But I have to tell you that this isn't the official position, which still advises diabetics to eat starchy foods regularly and without any restriction, i.e. over half a person's daily calorie intake is to be made up of these infamous 'slow sugars'. This advice is based on the fact that if we cut down on carbs, all we have left to eat is fats and proteins, and then it's harder to get patients to eat healthily. Which is true in part; however, the official guidance manages somewhere along the line to completely overlook the huge role that one particular food group could play, a group that alone could solve the problem – vegetables.

Vegetables are not starchy foods, although they do contain a small proportion of carbs. However, these carbs are in such low concentrations, are so entrapped in fibrous structures and drowned in so much water that their potential for causing any harm is negligible. Carb absorption is so sporadic that insulin does not even get activated.

Even if you're not trying to diet, if you think you need carbs for energy and you don't want to run the risk of gaining any weight, green vegetables are a fantastic, healthy source. Just think back to the hunter-gatherers, who had to undergo intense physical effort on a daily basis, and who nevertheless managed to survive by feeding off leaves and roots whenever the prey they hunted became scarce due to the long, cold winters.

So today, Saturday, you're allowed one portion of starchy foods, but the portion amount depends on the texture of the starchy food you opt for. Depending on whether it's lentils or mash, this portion may triple. Do bear this variation in mind, because later on when you have to keep the weight off, it'll help you work out just how friendly these different carbs are.

Which Starchy Foods Are You Allowed?

210g (7½oz) lentils, beans and chickpeas
To my mind, lentils are the least dangerous starchy food and this explains the nice large 210g (7½oz) portion. If you like lentils, you can treat yourself, and they'll leave you feeling really full and satisfied. They're a very useful

starchy food because of their good dose of high-quality fibre and not insignificant protein content.

I've grouped haricot beans (white beans) and chick-peas with lentils. Their sugar is absorbed at around the same rate and in the same concentration as lentils. However, not everyone enjoys their texture, flavour and palatability to quite the same extent.

200g (7oz) quinoa

Another food that comes to us from the Incas, like toma-toes and sweetcorn. Increasingly popular, quinoa can be easily found in supermarkets.

Like lentils, quinoa is high in protein and fibre and is one of the least fattening carbs. Many chefs who enjoy trying out new ingredients have come up with lots of tasty quinoa recipes.

190g (6½oz) pasta cooked al dente

This is a good-sized portion, so enjoy it. Eat your pasta al dente, i.e. not overcooked, because the more you cook pasta, the more you break down its resistance to being digested and assimilated. By doing this, you're doing the work your body is meant to do. From placing the pasta in your mouth to when it enters your bloodstream, diges-tion will be far quicker and so you'll secrete more insulin. Eating pasta al dente is far better.

Al dente is how the Italians, the pasta nation, have been cooking their pasta for centuries – not for nutritional reasons but because it tastes better and has a far better texture.

190g (6½oz) grilled corn on the cob

I'll take the opportunity here to speak about corn on the cob. It was a dietary staple of the Native Americans long before Columbus arrived. It's a favourite food with the American food-processing industry too, which turns it into a multitude of products. This provides us with a concrete example of the role that industry, and by extension the economy, plays in the food and nutrition sector.

So let me take you on a guided tour which you should find highly informative.

Pick a corn of cob from a field and if possible grill it on the same day. Given its texture and the time it takes to digest it, the glycaemic index is 36. What is the glycaemic index? It measures what takes place in the bloodstream once food has been ingested. Glycaemia is checked, which is the blood glucose content per litre. Normally, if you're not diabetic, your glycaemia will rise until it reaches a peak then once the insulin kicks in it will drop down again. Most importantly, the glycaemic index measures the rate at which glycaemia rises and the amount of insulin that is then released, and the weight gain this produces, which is what we're interested in. For fresh corn on the cob, a glycaemic index of 36 is a low index and close to that of lentils.

Take this corn cob, shell the maize and tin it in liquid where it will soak until sold and eaten. From 36 for fresh corn, the glycaemic index will shoot up to 50 for the tinned version, and what was a low index has now become an intermediate index, so you should go easy on tinned sweetcorn.

Next, take the corn and grind it until it turns into corn-flour powder. Just crushing the corn raises the glycaemic index to 70, so that you're now dealing with a fast carb that can be dangerous if you overindulge.

Now let's imagine that you make a dough by mixing this flour with water and that you feed this dough through rollers similar to ones that make paper. By now the corn's original structure has been completely broken down, there is no resistance, and a look through a microscope will reveal what remains – a nutritional desert. Depending on the country where it's produced, the index for this crushed dough will have rocketed to between 82 and 92, which is about as high as you can go.

So what do you end up with? A product that passes through your digestive tract like lightning, making your blood sugar level rise dramatically with a corresponding release of insulin, which is so violent that if this happens repeatedly it's likely to weaken your pancreas and tire it out. And, apart from putting on weight, if diabetes runs in your family you're likely to become diabetic.

And do you know what this rolled-out dough is used for? To make corn flakes, those lovely golden, crispy flakes that children adore and carry on eating when they grow up and which they then in turn feed to their own children.

170g (6oz) soft cooked pasta

As we've seen, if you cook pasta for long enough it softens, which cuts down the work your digestion should be carrying out. As a result the sugar in the pasta gets into your bloodstream more quickly and I think you know by now what happens next . . .

170g (6oz) brown rice

All types of rice have relatively fast penetrating sugars but because of its fibrous husk, it takes far longer to digest and assimilate brown rice. So that it passes through your system even more slowly, cook your rice with some vegetables and even a little minced meat or try it with crushed fish roe like the Cape Verdeans or with egg and low-fat ham like the Cantonese.

160g (5¾oz) tinned sweetcorn

I've just explained how tinned sweetcorn in liquid comes pre-digested and how the food-processing industry relieves you of this work. The aim is to make the corn easier to eat but also to make more money. Just as with white rice or white flour, the mechanization and processing facilities, as well as the canning process, lower production costs, but on the other hand they push up the price to the consumer. What the food-processing industry is doing is putting a premium on laziness. Refining foodstuffs for ease of use is an economic windfall to be sure, but a nightmare as far as nutrition is concerned. Industrial refining processes were developed after 1944; a time when being overweight did not yet occur in any population group.

150g (5½oz) white rice

I won't go over the lesson on texture and carb assimilation again; you see how once your rice is white the portion gets reduced.

140g (5oz) baked potato

The Frenchman Antoine Auguste Parmentier popularized potatoes at a time when wheat supplies in Europe were scarce, making it an expensive commodity. The huge advantage of the potato was that it gave manual workers loads of energy and very quickly. And fibre? You can see just how easy it is to cut a cooked potato in half and how its texture falls apart as you eat it. What all this means is quick entry into the bloodstream, insulin and fat.

80g (3oz) mashed potato

Once again, manufactured mashed potato flakes, so handy and quick, break down whatever resistance is left in the potato's texture, which compels me to restrict the portion weight for mash. But be aware that even with such a small dose, mashed potato can make you put on weight. So I'd strongly recommend you opt instead for the first starchy foods on the list – lentils, chickpeas and quinoa.

Which Starchy Food Should You Choose?

My recommendation is to start by selecting the one you'll enjoy – always go for what you enjoy! But if you have no particular preference, opt for lentils and quinoa, as they produce the least insulin and are therefore the ones that are less fattening.

Get into the habit of never eating any starchy or high-sugar food on its own. By combining them with other foods that take a long time to digest you will slow down absorption. The three best ways of slowing down sugar absorption is to eat vegetables, proteins and fats. You'll object and point out that fats are high in calories. This is true, but – I'll keep on telling you this, and I agree it's not easy to admit it when you've heard the very opposite – 'overweightness', obesity and diabetes are far more susceptible to carbs than to fats and proteins. This will come as a surprise, but 250g (9oz) of pasta is just as fattening eaten on its own as the same amount of pasta eaten with 30g (1oz) of minced beef. Although you've added some calories, the effect of these is offset because sugar absorption is slowed down and the amount of insulin secreted is reduced.

Oat Bran

The oat bran dose remains 1½ tablespoons, which is what you need to protect your weekend and make your oat bran galette.

Konjac

Again, it's the same prescription for konjac. Since starchy foods are introduced on Saturday you may feel tempted to cut down on your konjac. Please don't even contemplate this – you should do quite the reverse. So, if you've grown accustomed to konjac to the point where, for you, there's no real difference between them and traditional pasta, there's nothing to stop you from eating konjac instead of these starchy foods. This is only a suggestion and not an instruction; you're free to choose. Personally, since it's been possible to buy shiratakis with Bolognese sauce, we often eat them at home. I have to tell you that I really love pasta and I only really enjoy it if I get a proper plateful. What's more, if you substitute konjac for pasta you can add some cheese and a little butter. Don't forget that you can now buy konjac rice. At present I'm working with Japanese manufacturers to try to make konjac couscous, which should soon become available in the shops.

Saturday's Drink: Green Tea and Cayenne Pepper Infusion

As we're aiming to get through the weekend and at the same time keep risk to the minimum, I'm asking you to make your infusion today by increasing the dose as follows: 15–20g (½–¾oz) of green tea leaves or green tea pearls in 1 litre (1¾ pints) of water, add 2 pinches of cayenne pepper instead of one, 1 whole small lime and 4 teaspoons of sucralose. And as always remember the role that cold plays in thermogenesis and drink your infusion as chilled as possible in five portions spread throughout the day.

Exercise

Since Saturday and Sunday are in a weight-gaining phase, you'll need to take some precautions to avoid seeing the weekend finish in disaster.

So your instruction today is to walk not for half an hour but for one whole hour.

You can space this out and walk twice for 30 minutes or even go for three shorter 20-minute walks. The really important thing is that you walk as much as you can, immediately after you've had the meal containing the starchy foods. Try to visualize what's happening in your body: as long as the glucose provided by your meal hasn't yet been expelled from the bloodstream and turned into fat or glycogen, it remains exposed and vulnerable. So if you walk while you're still digesting, you'll burn it off more easily, which means you'll lower the insulin required to put it in quarantine. Think about this every time you eat a meal of fast carbs, or, better still, during the meal itself, just when you're being handed the serving bowl full of rice or pasta!

Your Diet Summary Sheet for Saturday

Today, on the first Saturday of your programme, you're allowed proteins, vegetables, fruit, two slices of bread, a portion of cheese and, at last, **one portion of starchy foods.**

Take great care to stick to the amount permitted for your starchy food. Use my whole description of them to help you.

Saturday is a day to relax, before you finally get Sunday's reward.

- Lean meats: veal, beef (except rib of beef and rib-eye steak), grilled or roasted without any fat

- Offal: liver, kidneys, and calf's and beef tongue (the tip)
- All fish: oily, lean, white, cooked and uncooked
- All seafood (shellfish and crustaceans)
- All poultry, except goose and duck, and without any skin
- Low-fat, cooked, sliced ham, chicken and turkey
- Eggs
- Vegetable proteins
- Fat-free dairy products
- 1.5 litres (2½ pints) of water (low sodium)
- An oat bran galette or 1½ tablespoons oat bran in milk, yoghurt or fromage frais
- Konjac
- A compulsory one-hour walk
- Your extras: coffee, tea, herbal teas, green tea with cayenne pepper, vinegars, seasonings, herbs, spices, gherkins, lemons, salt and mustard (in moderation)
- All cooked and uncooked vegetables
- One portion of fruit, except bananas, grapes, dried fruit such as dried apricots and prunes, and oleaginous fruits like walnuts, almonds, peanuts, pistachios and other nuts
- Two slices of wholegrain or wholemeal bread
- One portion of hard or soft rind cheese, less than 50% fat
- The permitted amount of one portion of starchy food (lentils, beans, chickpeas, quinoa, al dente or soft pasta, grilled corn on the cob or tinned sweetcorn, white or brown rice, baked or mashed potatoes)

AND NOTHING ELSE!

DAILY RECIPES

PROTEIN, VEGETABLE, FRUIT, BREAD, CHEESE AND STARCHY FOOD RECIPES FOR **SATURDAY**

(and for Sunday too)

CHICKEN LIVER RISOTTO

(4 servings)
Preparation time: 20 minutes
Cooking time: 25 minutes

1 large onion, finely chopped
2 garlic cloves, finely chopped
200g (7oz) Arborio rice
1 litre (1¾ pints) hot chicken stock, fat skimmed off
150g (5½oz) virtually fat-free quark
400g (14oz) chicken livers, cut into strips
Raspberry vinegar
Freshly ground black pepper

Sweat the onion and garlic in a high-sided non-stick frying pan over a medium heat without any fat. Add the rice and toast it for 1 minute, stirring all the time, then gradually work in the chicken stock. Wait for each ladleful to be absorbed before adding the next one. The rice should be cooked but still slightly firm.

When ready, remove from the heat and stir in the quark.

Meanwhile, in another non-stick frying pan, fry the chicken livers without any fat for 4–5 minutes over a fairly high heat. Remove the pan from the heat, pour in a generous dash of raspberry vinegar then add some freshly ground black pepper.

Serve the risotto surrounded by the chicken livers.

WHOLEWHEAT PASTA WITH GARLIC, BRESAOLA AND MATURE MIMOLETTE

(4 servings)
Preparation time: 15 minutes
Cooking time: 10 minutes

250g (9oz) wholewheat pasta shells (or wholewheat fusilli)
6 garlic cloves, finely chopped
10 slices of bresaola, cut into small pieces
2 egg yolks
160g (5¾oz) mature Mimolette cheese (or mature cheddar), shaved
Salt and black pepper

Bring a large saucepan of salted water to the boil, add the pasta shells and cook for 7 minutes – the pasta should be al dente.

Meanwhile, heat some water in the bottom of a non-stick frying pan and fry the garlic and bresaola over a high heat, stirring all the time. Remove the pan from the heat.

Drain the pasta and rinse in cold water. Place the frying pan with the garlic and bresaola back over a gentle heat and add the pasta shells. Heat through for 2 minutes, stirring all the time. Add the egg yolks and cheese and season with salt and black pepper. Stir well and divide the pasta between 4 plates. Serve piping hot.

KONJAC SPINACH TAGLIATELLE WITH BROAD BEANS

(4 servings)
Preparation time: 15 minutes
Cooking time: 20 minutes

Frozen broad beans are widely available in super-markets and very handy for cooking. Cumin with broad beans is a delightful combination.

1 litre (1¾ pints) chicken stock, made with a salt-reduced stock cube
200g (7oz) frozen broad beans (double podded)
2 small onions, finely chopped

250g (9oz) tomatoes, peeled and cut into strips
2 packets of Dukan Diet konjac spinach tagliatelle
80g (3oz) Parmesan cheese, grated
Salt and cumin

Bring the stock to the boil in a saucepan. Add the broad beans, a pinch of salt and some cumin and leave to cook for 5 minutes. Stir in the onions and cook over a gentle heat for a further 5 minutes.

Add the tomatoes to the saucepan and continue cooking for at least another 5 minutes, stirring at regular intervals, to reduce the sauce down to the desired consistency (if necessary, drain off any excess liquid). Once the sauce is ready, set aside and keep warm.

Rinse the konjac spinach tagliatelle. Add the tagliatelle to a large saucepan of boiling salted water and cook for 2 minutes. Rinse the tagliatelle, drain well and stir in the tomato and broad bean sauce. Serve piping hot, with the grated Parmesan sprinkled over.

DOUBLE SALMON TARTARE
WITH RED QUINOA

(4 servings)
Preparation time: 20 minutes
Cooking time: 20 minutes

1 vegetable stock cube
130g (4¾oz) red quinoa, rinsed
1 teaspoon chopped dill
100g (3½oz) fat-free cottage cheese
200g (7oz) fresh salmon fillet, skin and bones removed
2 slices of smoked salmon
½ shallot, finely chopped
Juice of 1 lemon, plus lemon quarters to serve
1 teaspoon finely chopped chives
Salt and black pepper

Fill a large saucepan with cold water, crumble in the vegetable stock cube and add the quinoa. Bring to the boil and cook for 20 minutes over a gentle heat, until the small seeds split. Turn the heat off, cover and leave to swell for 6 minutes. Season sparingly with salt and black pepper. Divide the quinoa between 4 glass dishes.

Stir the dill into the cottage cheese. Season lightly with salt, add some black pepper and spoon a layer over the red quinoa in the dishes.

Using a very sharp knife, cut the raw salmon and the smoked salmon into small cubes. Add the shallot and the lemon juice. Mix together and spoon on to the layer of cottage cheese. Sprinkle over the chopped chives and place a lemon quarter on top of each dish.

Serve well chilled.

QUINOA AND BRESAOLA TIMBALES

(4 servings)
Preparation time: 20 minutes
Cooking time: 20 minutes + at least 2 hours chilling

If you can't refrigerate the timbales for 2 hours, just put them in the freezer for 20 minutes before turning them out.

150g (5½oz) quinoa, rinsed
300ml (10fl oz) chicken stock
6 portions virtually fat-free quark with chopped garlic and herbs
1 teaspoon sherry vinegar
2 tomatoes, deseeded and diced
8 thin slices of bresaola, cut into strips
Freshly ground black pepper
Rocket leaves, to serve

Put the quinoa in a saucepan with the stock and bring to the boil. Cover and simmer over a gentle heat for about 20 minutes. The stock should be completely absorbed. Remove the pan from the heat and leave to cool down.

Stir the quark into the quinoa, add the sherry vinegar and season with freshly ground black pepper. Add the tomato and bresaola. Stir all the ingredients together carefully.

Line 4 ramekin dishes with cling film. Divide the mixture between them, pressing it down into the dishes a little. Refrigerate for at least 2 hours.

When you are ready to serve, carefully ease the timbales out on to plates and arrange the rocket leaves around them.

TANDOORI CHICKEN WITH
RED LENTIL DHAL

(4 servings)
Preparation time: 40 minutes + overnight marinating
Cooking time: 30 minutes

For the tandoori chicken:
4 chicken breasts, cut into chunks
Juice of 1 lime
150g (5½oz) fat-free natural yoghurt
4 garlic cloves, crushed
3cm (1¼in) piece of fresh ginger, finely chopped
4 tablespoons tandoori spice mixture, powder or paste
Salt and black pepper
For the lentil dhal:
2 onions, finely chopped
4 garlic cloves, crushed

2 teaspoons curry paste or powder
1 teaspoon cumin
2 pinches of cayenne pepper
½ teaspoon cinnamon
2 teaspoons ground coriander
4 cardamom pods
2 tomatoes, deseeded and diced
280g (10oz) red lentils, rinsed
Juice of 1 lemon
Fresh coriander, finely chopped

Place the chicken in a large bowl, season with salt and black pepper and pour over the lime juice. Stir well so that the chicken is well coated and leave to marinate in the fridge for 1 hour. Mix together the yoghurt, garlic, ginger and tandoori spices. Add to the chicken and stir thoroughly. Leave to marinate in the fridge overnight.

The following day, cook the chicken in a frying pan for 12–15 minutes. Keep a careful eye on the pan and if necessary pour in some marinade. When cooked through, set the chicken aside and keep warm.

Meanwhile, make the dhal. Fry the onions and garlic in a little water in a high-sided frying pan. Add the curry paste or powder, cumin, cayenne pepper, cinnamon, ground coriander and cardamom and fry for a further 2 minutes. Next add the tomatoes and soften for 2 minutes. Finally add the red lentils, dry-fry them for 2 minutes and then cover with 500ml (18fl oz) of water.

Bring to the boil, cover and cook for 15–20 minutes over a low heat. The dhal is ready once the lentils start to become really tender. Stir in the lemon juice and sprinkle with the chopped coriander. Serve with the tandoori chicken.

BEEF CARPACCIO WITH CHICKPEAS

(4 servings)
Preparation time: 15 minutes + 30 minutes chilling
No cooking required

Juice of 3 lemons
8 slices of rump steak, very thinly sliced
840g tinned chickpeas
Cumin
Salt and black pepper

Make a dressing by mixing the lemon juice with some salt and black pepper.

Arrange the steak slices on 4 plates and pour over the dressing. Cover the carpaccio with the chickpeas and sprinkle over some cumin. Cover the plates with cling film and refrigerate for 30 minutes before serving.

DUKAN-STYLE RACLETTE

(4 servings)
Preparation time: 20 minutes
Cooking time: 30 minutes

A raclette in a diet book?! Well, yes – proof if any were needed that the Nutritional Staircase doesn't stop you from enjoying food with friends, since you're even allowed 'raclette evenings'.

560g (1lb 4¼oz) potatoes, scrubbed
200g (7oz) bresaola
160g (5¾oz) raclette cheese, thinly sliced
320g (11¼oz) crème fraîche
Silverskin or small pickled onions
Cornichons

Boil the potatoes in a large saucepan of salted water for about 20 minutes. Check they are ready by inserting the tip of a knife – it should go in easily. Keep warm.

Arrange the bresaola slices on a serving platter. Switch on the raclette machine if you have one.

Melt the cheese on the raclette machine or in a microwave for 30 seconds.

Place a portion of raclette cheese on each person's plate, and serve the crème fraîche, onions and cornichons in small individual bowls.

Enjoy with the cooked potatoes, bresaola, crème fraîche and pickles.

Sunday

THE LEITMOTIF
Monday for what's vital
Tuesday for what's essential
Wednesday for what's important
Thursday for what's useful
Friday for what's smooth and creamy
Saturday for energy
and Sunday for freedom!

Sunday and Monday are poles apart nutritionally speaking and food-wise, but they are also, of course, next to one another. On the one hand, as you climb up the Nutritional Staircase, Sunday is the day that is most different from Monday because of the wide range of foods you're now free to eat. Sunday is enriched by the week's succession of food groups and crowned by its celebration meal. On the other hand, although totally opposed these two days border one another and complement each other. And this is significant. There's a German proverb that says 'the trees don't grow up to the sky'. With a programme designed to make you lose weight, you know that the free rein has to come to an end.

Today it's Sunday and, in line with tradition, this is a day for celebration, so relax and make the most of it without feeling any guilt. Tomorrow it'll be Monday, the buffer day that's there to set the counter back to zero.

You see, I've constructed my Nutritional Staircase so that, as you climb up it, there's:

- A FUN ELEMENT, each day bringing a new reward.
- A DIDACTIC ELEMENT, providing a path so you learn about the importance of a food group according to when it joins the path.
- AND YOU'RE OFFERED PROTECTION with the return of Monday and Tuesday, to keep you safe and prevent your body from profiting all it can from the freedom of the weekend.

Those who've followed the second front have enjoyed this seven-day cycle. It appeals to the particular psychology of food control alongside a reward structure, with cycles for enjoyment and restoring control, which are both equally sought after. And they also liked the fact that this weekly routine – which goes from what is most necessary to what is most gratifying – created simple markers for them and a clear value hierarchy for the foods as they are gradually introduced.

Step by step, the Nutritional Staircase has taught you the value and importance of foods. The repetition of this hierarchy of values sets up new messages and new circuits in your brain, which over time become virtuous reflex actions or, in other words, good habits.

This Sunday, you are allowed:

- all Monday's high-protein foods
- vegetables
- fruit
- two slices of wholegrain or wholemeal bread
- a portion of hard cheese
- and the famous **celebration meal**, the high point of your week.

Do remember that this is a meal and not a whole day; you have your celebration meal either for lunch or supper.

The starchy food portion allowed for Saturday cannot be added to the celebration meal as this would be too much, but it can form part of it – either as a main course such as tuna paella, seafood pasta, pizza, cassoulet or Portuguese Feijoada (a meat and bean stew), or as the accompaniment to your meat or fish (rice, quinoa or lentils).

What Is a Celebration Meal Exactly?

Firstly, it must be thought of as a celebration. It's a pleasure that's there to reward you for getting to the end of the week. You mustn't eat it thinking you're getting your own back, as the bitterness of revenge would dispel all the joy.

I designed and developed this second front so that it would have a breathing space.

The start to the week is strong, very strong even, but you know that it'll only last a single day. We're all prepared to make this effort, especially when it pays off. Many people who follow my second front have even asked me if they could extend Monday into Tuesday evening.

You start off by breathing in on Monday and carrying on with almost as much vigour on Tuesday. This tapers off slightly on Wednesday and ends on Thursday. Friday is the turning point, perfectly balanced, and on Saturday and Sunday you can breathe out again. Each day is different from the one before, bringing something new, its own contribution and reward. Sunday brings up the rear by allowing you EVERYTHING you want in one meal.

Start with a **first course**, whatever you like. You fancy a slice of foie gras? You can have it, or some Parma ham, an avocado salad or guacamole. Let loose your imagination – I'll help you!

What you have for your **main course** is also totally up to you; choose whatever takes your fancy. Couscous? Cassoulet? Paella? Rib steak with chanterelle mushroom spaghetti and so on. I could carry on over thousands of pages as we've reached another dimension – we're now talking about pure pleasure.

And your **dessert**? Here again you're free to choose. If you don't have a sweet tooth, you could just as easily have cheese instead.

And to crown it all, you're allowed one glass of wine, of whatever type or colour you wish. Take a standard glass and fill it up as you want, but always keep to a centimetre from the top.

If you don't drink, obviously you shouldn't force yourself; it's something you're allowed to have but it's not obligatory! The same goes for the actual celebration meal. It's part of the rules of the game, but if you're not bothered about it then you can decide what to do.

However, as far as quantities are concerned there are limits. Whether it's your starter, main course or pudding, you must base your portion size on what you'd be served in a restaurant. Whether you're at home or with friends, the instruction is clear and uncompromising: you do just as you would in a restaurant and **you never take seconds of any course.**

Oat Bran

Take care, the one day you mustn't forget your oat bran is Sunday. The dose remains the same. Try and stick to your galette with egg white and fromage frais as proteins always help you get through tricky times.

Konjac

Again, you need to stick to your konjac. It provides a counterbalance to this apex day and is all the easier because there's nothing punitive about konjac. Konjac could even be part of your celebration meal.

I'd like to talk to you about anatomy and some common sense.

Our stomach is a hollow, muscular organ which, when

full, has an average volume of 2 litres (3½ pints), depending on the person's size, age and appetite.

This is a lot and a little. A lot if you fill it with fatty and especially sugary foods, but it's a little if you fill it with vegetables, protein foods and water. Two large glasses of water and already that's almost half a litre. Two large tomatoes or chicories and there's another half-litre, and if you add a nice chicken drumstick you've got another 300–400g (10½–14oz). We've already got to 1.4 litres (2½ pints) or 1 kilo (2lb 4oz). If you then include a little oat bran and some konjac, you're filling your stomach up some more.

As you absorb these foods, each mouthful, each time you chew, each sensation perceived by your tongue, palate and the mucous membranes in your cheeks, each time you swallow and each smell are all signals that combine and get sent to your brain – they show up on a gauge that tells your brain just how full your stomach is.

As this gauge gradually rises, what is called 'automatic satiety' develops, and usually once the stomach is two-thirds full, we no longer have an intense appetite. Yet, it's precisely at this moment that starchy foods appear and immediately after them cheese and pudding, all dangers to be avoided.

The hunter-gatherers had to be really racked by hunger to want to go off and hunt, to brave danger and ferocious animals just to find something to survive. They used up energy as they walked miles to glean some sustenance. And as soon as they felt full up, they would stop eating. Whereas the way we live nowadays is in contradiction to this overpowering survival programming. Because we have abundant food all around us, the way we feel hunger and satiety is somewhat disrupted. At any time we can eat sugars that are so addictive and fatty foods that are so tasty. Therefore, in order to withstand such temptation, we need to fill ourselves up and automatically satisfy our appetite.

Store away this piece of strategic information, as it'll help you work out how best to structure your mealtimes, especially when you're in stabilization. It's not about laying down rules, but simply a way for you to structure your eating. Once I'm no longer there to supervise you, it can work away on its own.

Sunday's Drink: Green Tea and Cayenne Pepper Infusion

• Keep to yesterday's instructions with the increased dose for the weekend: 1 litre (1¾ pints) of water, 15–20g (½–¾oz) of green tea leaves or green tea pearls, 2 pinches of cayenne pepper, the juice of 1 small lime and 4 teaspoons of sucralose. Drink your infusion in five portions spread over the day and as cold as possible.

Exercise

• Your instructions are the same as for Saturday – please go walking for an hour. If you wish, you can split this over two or even three sessions, but what I'm most concerned about is that at least some of this walking takes place after your celebration meal. After 30 minutes the sugar reaches your bloodstream and each step you take means you stop a little sugar from getting stored away as fat in your stomach or on your hips.

My Final Tips

- Weigh yourself every morning before you eat so that you can plot a graph of your weight. Each time you notice a loss, however tiny it may be, this will lift your spirits and inspire you to do even better; this is called 'joining the winning side'!
- If you notice any weight gain this will also help you get back on track.
- Don't forget that if you've just lapsed badly and want to neutralize the effects, then have a protein day the next day instead of what was scheduled, and then continue climbing the Staircase the day after.
- For example, Wednesday is a Proteins + Vegetables + Fruit day. Imagine that you went completely off course. The following day, Thursday, instead of moving into the Thursday cycle and adding two slices of bread, you have pure proteins and then the following day, Friday, you go back to your normal Friday with fruit, bread and cheese.
- Finally, I'd advise you to plot your weight using some graph paper so that you can compare your progress from week to week.
- If you can, subscribe to personalized coaching on the internet, as it's a great way to help you succeed.

- If your budget is tight, use frozen foods. You can buy very high-quality vegetables, fruit and fish.

The Carbs Reflex

During the first four days of your weight-loss period, from Monday to Thursday, avoid all sugar entirely. Avoid white flour and especially any starchy foods made from both sugar and flour.

And looking forwards to the future, try to preserve a way of thinking that will protect you from growing over-weight and putting the pounds back on, i.e. the 'carbs reflex'.

Read the food labels; you'll see how many calories there are and the percentage of proteins and fats. This information is useful and can guide you. But for your weight in the future, the key detail is what you'll find on the lines: 'Carbohydrates' and 'of which sugars'. I spoke to you about this at the start of your Nutritional Staircase.

However, I'm now going to clarify this further and make an important point.

To understand what is at stake here, you need to remember that **not all carbs have the same glycaemic index**. I've told you how starchy foods have different glycaemic indexes, and that you should go for lentils or quinoa instead of white rice. Carbs are not digested or assimilated at the same speed nor are they equally adipogenous (fat producing). Refined sugar, white flour, honey and corn flakes get absorbed ultra-rapidly. Let's go back to the line 'of which sugars': this is pure refined sugar, the

273

most invasive of all carbs, which triggers the greatest insulin secretion and causes the greatest transformation into fat.

Be very wary of any product, even if sold with the reassuring words 'nutritional' or 'health food', that displays on the 'of which sugars' line more than 7–8g of pure sugar – 20g will very soon be turned into 10g of your fat. And once it has settled, it's so much more difficult to shift than if you'd never put it on in the first place.

What's more, we now have positive proof that sugar is addictive. The sensations produced by sugar follow the same reward circuits in the brain as those that treat the hardest drugs.

At the risk of boring you, I've stressed time and again how sugar causes weight problems. I've repeated myself because I'm neither a novelist nor an essayist but a doctor. And by reiterating ideas I have, I hope, made you aware that you must cut down your carb intake permanently. In my heart and soul, I believe that your health and life expectancy are at issue here, as well as of course the weight you're currently losing and that you want to maintain afterwards. So please don't blame me for this but rather take it as proof of my friendship and kindness towards you. And should I have succeeded in persuading you of the carbs/insulin argument, please learn to be vigilant and adopt the carbs reflex. Stick with it and, most importantly, stick by it after you've lost weight – it'll be the spearhead for your stabilization.

Your Diet Summary Sheet for Sunday

Today, on the first Sunday of your programme, you keep all Monday's high-protein foods and to them you add vegetables, fruit, your two slices of bread and one portion of cheese.

However, Sunday is also a day of celebration – so you're allowed one **celebration meal**. Remember – this is just a single meal, either lunch or dinner, and not the whole day!

- Lean meats: veal, beef (except rib of beef and rib-eye steak), grilled or roasted without any fat
- Offal: liver, kidneys, and calf's and beef tongue (the tip)
- All fish: oily, lean, white, cooked and uncooked
- All seafood (shellfish and crustaceans)
- All poultry, except goose and duck, and without any skin
- Low-fat, cooked, sliced ham, chicken and turkey
- Eggs
- Vegetable proteins
- Fat-free dairy products
- 1.5 litres (2½ pints) of water (low sodium)
- An oat bran galette or 1½ tablespoons oat bran in milk, yoghurt or fromage frais
- Konjac
- A compulsory one-hour walk
- Your extras: coffee, tea, herbal teas, green tea with cayenne pepper, vinegars, seasonings, herbs, spices, gherkins, lemons, salt and mustard (in moderation)

- All cooked and uncooked vegetables
- One portion of fruit, except bananas, grapes, dried fruit such as dried apricots and prunes, and oleaginous fruits like walnuts, almonds, peanuts, pistachios and other nuts
- Two slices of wholegrain or wholemeal bread
- One portion of hard or soft rind cheese, less than 50% fat
- Included in the celebration meal are: one portion of starchy foods in the permitted quantities (lentils, beans, chickpeas, quinoa, al dente or soft pasta, grilled corn on the cob or tinned sweetcorn, white or brown rice, baked or mashed potatoes)
- One celebration meal with a starter, main course and dessert – you can even pour yourself a glass of wine!

DAILY RECIPES

RECIPES FOR **SUNDAY**

(all celebration meal recipes only)

'ASSIETTE GOURMANDE'

(4 servings)
Preparation time: 10 minutes
No cooking required

If you cannot find these exact ingredients, substitute with alternatives of your choice but keep to these quantities.

150g (5½oz) duck pâté
Fleur de sel or sea salt flakes
8 chives, chopped
100g (3½oz) fig and onion compote
100g (3½oz) smoked goose or duck breast, sliced
Seasonal green salad
4 slices of gingerbread

Dip a sharp knife in hot water and use it to divide the pâté into 4 equal slices. Arrange the pâté on 4 plates and scatter over a little sea salt and some chopped chives. Spoon some compote into 4 tiny pots and place one on each plate.

Spread the goose breast slices in a fan shape around the pâté and add a little green salad as an accompaniment, drizzled with some dressing of your choice.

Toast the gingerbread. Cut the slices into long strips, arranging half on the plate and the rest on top of the tiny pots of compote.

LAMB MEATLOAF

(4 servings)
Preparation time: 15 minutes + 30 minutes chilling
Cooking time: 45 minutes + 10 minutes resting

3 heads of garlic
600g (1lb 5oz) minced lamb
A dash of milk
2 tablespoons breadcrumbs
2 eggs
Some thyme leaves
A knob of butter
Fleur de sel or sea salt flakes and black pepper
1 sachet of quick-cook couscous
1 handful of raisins
1 handful of pine nuts
1 tablespoon olive oil
100ml (3½fl oz) veal (or lamb) stock

Sunday

Preheat the oven to 180°C/350°F/Gas 4.

Remove all the cloves from the heads of garlic and cook them in a pan of boiling salted water for 10 minutes without peeling them, then drain.

In a large bowl, knead together the lamb, milk, breadcrumbs, eggs, thyme and a little sea salt. Leave to rest in the fridge for 30 minutes then shape the mixture into a loaf. Melt the knob of butter in an ovenproof dish. Place the meatloaf in the dish, arrange the garlic cloves all around it and sprinkle all over with some water. Bake in the preheated oven for 45 minutes.

Meanwhile, 10 minutes before the meatloaf is ready, soak the raisins in a bowl of water. Cook the couscous according to the packet instructions. Mix in the raisins, pine nuts and olive oil.

Remove the meatloaf from the oven and leave it to rest for 10 minutes. Pour the stock into the dish and return to the heat to reduce by half.

Serve the meatloaf with the garlic cloves arranged around it, accompanied by the couscous and the sauce.

BEEF TOURNEDOS ROSSINI

(4 servings)
Preparation time: 20 minutes
Cooking time: 10 minutes

4 slices of white sandwich bread
4 × 150g tournedos
2 tablespoons oil
2 tablespoons butter
4 medallions of duck pâté, 5mm (¼in) thick
I small glass of Madeira or port
300ml (10fl oz) veal stock
Thin shavings of black truffles (optional)
Fleur de sel or sea salt flakes and freshly ground 5
peppercorn mix

Toast the sandwich bread. Using a pastry cutter, cut out circles the same size as the tournedos (or slightly larger).

Cover 2 plates with aluminium foil. Heat the oil and butter in a frying pan then fry the tournedos for 3–4 minutes on each side (depending on how well done you like your steak). Season with salt and ground peppercorn mix. When cooked, trim off any fat. Set aside on a foil-covered plate and keep warm.

Next, fry the pâté for 2 minutes, making sure that it remains nice and pink on the inside. Set aside on the second foil-covered plate and keep warm.

Deglaze the bottom of the frying pan with the Madeira or port and add the veal stock. Stir and cook to reduce the sauce.

Arrange the toast circles on 4 plates. Spoon over some of the hot sauce, place a warm tournedos on top, followed by the pâté and finish off with the truffle shavings, if using. Pour over more of the hot sauce and serve straightaway.

JAPANESE-STYLE CHOCOLATE FONDANT

(4 servings)
Preparation time: 15 minutes
Cooking time: 20 minutes

If you don't have any Asian grocery stores nearby, you can buy wasabi in supermarkets. If you don't like the taste, replace it with a teaspoon of coffee.

1 teaspoon wasabi
3 eggs + 2 egg whites
1 pinch of salt
200g (7oz) dark chocolate (minimum 70% cocoa solids)
100g (3½oz) butter, cubed
100g (3½oz) sugar (or 3 tablespoons agave syrup)
60g (2¼oz) flour

Dilute the wasabi in a tablespoon of warm water so that it is easy to use. Preheat the oven to 160°C/325°F/ Gas 3.

Break the whole eggs and separate the yolks from the whites. Whisk all the whites with the salt until nice and stiff.

Break the chocolate into a small heatproof bowl with a little water. Set the bowl over a saucepan of gently simmering water to melt the chocolate. Add the butter and melt it with the chocolate. Remove from the heat and stir in the wasabi and then the sugar. Stir to mix thoroughly.

Gradually add in the egg yolks and flour, stirring all the time so that the mixture is nice and smooth. Carefully fold in the egg whites and pour the mixture into a mould. Bake in the preheated oven for 20 minutes, keeping a careful eye on it to check when it is ready.

CHOCOLATE MOUSSE WITH STEM GINGER AND CANDIED ORANGE PEEL

(4 servings)
Preparation time: 15 minutes
Cooking time: 5 minutes + 3 hours chilling

8 strips of candied orange peel
150g (5½oz) dark chocolate (minimum 70% cocoa solids)
2 tablespoons ginger liqueur (optional)
4 eggs
60g (2¼oz) stem ginger, chopped
1 pinch of salt

Chop 4 of the candied orange peel strips into tiny pieces.

Melt the chocolate in a bowl set over a saucepan of gently simmering water for about 5 minutes. Add the ginger liqueur.

Break the eggs, separating the whites from the yolks.

Pour the melted chocolate over the egg yolks and stir together vigorously. Add three-quarters of the chopped stem ginger.

Whisk the egg whites with the salt until stiff. Carefully fold the egg whites into the chocolate mixture. Pour the mousse into 4 large sundae dishes and refrigerate for at least 3 hours.

When you are ready to serve, sprinkle the remaining pieces of ginger over the mousses and decorate each one with a strip of candied orange peel.

Menu Ideas

Winter Menu

	MONDAY	TUESDAY	WEDNESDAY
	Pure Proteins	**Proteins Vegetables**	**Proteins Vegetables Fruit**
Breakfast	Fat-free fromage frais Turkey breast **Oat bran galette (p143)**	Fat-free cottage cheese **Oat bran galette (p143)** Home-made rhubarb compote	Home-made egg custard ½ grapefruit Oat bran muffin
Lunch	Bresaola slices **Chicken and turmeric loaf (p144)** Home-made egg custard, flavour of your choice	Grated carrot salad **Konjac shirataki noodles with Bolognese sauce (p171)** Fat-free strawberry-flavoured yoghurt	Chicory salad Skirt of beef with shallots French beans Fat-free cottage cheese
Snack	Fat-free fromage frais with cinnamon	Fat-free cottage cheese	Fat-free coconut-flavoured yoghurt
Dinner	Prawns Fried scallops Konjac shirataki noodles with ginger and soy sauce Dukan mocha meringues	Cauliflower cream soup with cumin **Asparagus and bresaola rolls with a herb salad (p170)** Home-made floating meringues	Beetroot and lamb's lettuce salad Finnan haddock fillet, lemony fromage frais sauce Plain sauerkraut Bitter almond milky jelly

Winter Menu

THURSDAY	FRIDAY	SATURDAY	SUNDAY
Proteins **Vegetables** **Fruit Bread**	**Proteins** **Vegetables Fruit** **Bread Cheese**	**Proteins** **Vegetables Fruit** **Bread Cheese** **Starchy Foods**	**Day with a celebration meal**
50g (1¾ oz) toasted wholemeal bread Fat-free fromage frais Home-made rhubarb compote	**Oat bran galette (p143)** Fat-free cottage cheese 1 soft-boiled egg 25g (1oz) wholemeal bread	50g (1¾oz) toasted wholemeal bread Fat-free fromage frais with cinnamon Home-made rhubarb compote	**Oat bran galette (p143)** Fat-free cottage cheese Home-made rhubarb compote
Dukan egg mayonnaise Roast chicken Provençal tomatoes Fat-free lemon-flavoured yoghurt	Dukan leeks in vinaigrette Fried veal escalope with lemon Braised chicory 40g (1½ oz) goat's cheese Fat-free honey-flavoured yoghurt	Crab and smoked salmon millefeuille **Konjac spinach tagliatelle with broad beans (p256)** Home-made egg custard, flavour of your choice	Prawn avocado with cocktail sauce **Beef tournedos Rossini (p280)** French beans and potato gratin dauphinoise Pear and chocolate crumble
Virtually fat-free quark Mandarin	25g (1oz) wholemeal bread Virtually fat-free quark	**Oat bran galette (p143)**	Home-made egg custard, flavour of your choice
Tuna mousse **Scallops with spicy oranges (p189)** Steamed fennel Home-made agar-agar crème caramel	Pumpkin and quark soup Fillet of salmon Mashed carrot and celeriac duo **Citrus syllabub (p197)**	Beetroot and lamb's lettuce salad Beef on a string with baby vegetables 40g (1½oz) Comté cheese Baked apple	Summer vegetable soup **Sardinian bruschetta, (p219)** tomato salad 40g (1½oz) pecorino cheese Home-made quince compote

Spring Menu

	MONDAY	TUESDAY	WEDNESDAY
	Pure Proteins	Proteins Vegetables	Proteins Vegetables Fruit
Breakfast	Fat-free fromage frais 1 soft-boiled egg **Oat bran galette (p143)**	Fat-free cottage cheese **Oat bran galette (p143)**	Home-made egg custard ½ small melon Oat bran muffin
Lunch	Tuna spread with preserved lemon Salmon sashimi Konjac shirataki noodles with ginger and soy sauce Fat-free coconut-flavoured yoghurt	Sliced cooked ham or turkey **Herb salad quartet with Saint-Pierrelin on toast (p212)** Fat-free lemon-flavoured yoghurt	Tomato and basil salad Skirt of beef with shallots Steamed courgettes ½ 1% fat Saint-Pierrelin or virtually fat-free quark
Snack	Fat-free cottage cheese with cinnamon	Fat-free coconut-flavoured yoghurt	1 hard-boiled egg Fat-free yoghurt
Dinner	Bresaola and virtually fat-free quark rolls Thyme and lemon veal escalope Vanilla fromage frais mousse	Vichy carrots with cumin Fresh herb omelette and salad **Rhubarb meringue compote (p176)**	Steamed artichoke with Maya salad dressing Salmon fillet, cooked on one side, with green asparagus Home-made coffee and bitter almond mousse

Spring Menu

THURSDAY	FRIDAY	SATURDAY	SUNDAY
Proteins Vegetables Fruit Bread	**Proteins Vegetables Fruit Bread Cheese**	**Proteins Vegetables Fruit Bread Cheese Starchy Foods**	**Day with a celebration meal**
50g (1¾oz) toasted wholemeal bread Fat-free fromage frais Home-made rhubarb compote	**Oat bran galette with cocoa (p143)** Fat-free cottage cheese 1 soft-boiled egg	**Oat bran galette (p143)** Fat-free fromage frais with cinnamon Home-made rhubarb compote	**Oat bran galette (p143)** 2 kiwis Fat-free cottage cheese
Lemony cucumber sticks Roast chicken French beans Fat-free strawberry-flavoured yoghurt	Seafood sticks **Tuna Provençal slices (p214)** 40g (1½oz) fruity Gouda	Raita salad with cucumber, garlic and yoghurt **Steak marinated in balsamic vinegar and mustard (p147)** Spinach Virtually fat-free quark	Assortment of Greek mezze: taramasalata, mushrooms, red peppers, tzatziki **Lamb meatloaf (p278)** Istanbul Muhallebi custard
Virtually fat-free quark **Oat bran galette (p143)**	Fat-free vanilla-flavoured yoghurt	Fat-free coconut-flavoured yoghurt 50g (1¾oz) wholemeal bread	Virtually fat-free quark
Beetroot and lamb's lettuce salad Vegetarian springtime stir-fry: vegetables, tofu, fat-free quark, pepper and pink peppercorns **Vanilla cheesecake with raspberry coulis (p193)**	Vegetable dip: carrots, cauliflower, cherry tomatoes with fat-free fromage frais and fresh chopped herbs **Sole, mango and fennel parcels** Cocoa ice cream with fresh raspberries (p191)	Finely chopped fennel salad with lemon **Wholewheat pasta shells with garlic, bresaola and mature Mimolette (p255)** Pineapple carpaccio	**Mediterranean slices (p218)** Mixed grill kebabs Baked tomatoes Home-made egg custard, flavour of your choice

Summer Menu

	MONDAY	TUESDAY	WEDNESDAY
	Pure Proteins	Proteins Vegetables	Proteins Vegetables Fruit
Breakfast	Fat-free fromage frais Turkey breast **Oat bran galette (p143)**	Fat-free cottage cheese **Oat bran galette (p143)** Home-made rhubarb compote	Home-made egg custard ½ small melon Oat bran muffin
Lunch	Tuna and quark mousse Seafood platter: prawns, mussels, marinated fish, scallops Fat-free vanilla-flavoured yoghurt	Gazpacho Big Niçoise salad with Maya salad dressing Fat-free lemon-flavoured yoghurt	Beetroot and cucumber salad Beef burger French beans ½ 1% fat Saint-Pierrelin or virtually fat-free quark
Snack	Fat-free cottage cheese with cinnamon	Fat-free coconut-flavoured yoghurt	1 hard-boiled egg Fat-free yoghurt
Dinner	Beef carpaccio, balsamic and basil vinaigrette **Crusty, spicy turkey strips (p290)** Dukan floating islands	Grated celeriac with Dukan mayonnaise Seared tuna steak, cooked on one side only, basil fromage frais sauce and Provençal tomatoes Home-made mint tea sorbet	Bresaola and quark rolls Roast chicken Mixed fried vegetables Home-made fat-free yoghurt ice-cream

Summer Menu

THURSDAY	FRIDAY	SATURDAY	SUNDAY
Proteins Vegetables Fruit Bread	**Proteins Vegetables Fruit Bread Cheese**	**Proteins Vegetables Fruit Bread Cheese Starchy Foods**	**Day with a celebration meal**
50g (1¾oz) toasted wholemeal bread Fat-free fromage frais Home-made rhubarb compote	50g (1¾oz) toasted wholemeal bread Fat-free cottage cheese 1 soft-boiled egg	**Oat bran galette (p143)** Fat-free fromage frais with cinnamon Home-made rhubarb compote	**Oat bran galette (p143)** ½ mango Fat-free cottage cheese
Radishes with salt Grilled turkey escalope and fried courgettes Smoothie: ¼ melon, fat-free creamy yoghurt and ice cubes	Tomato and basil salad **Beef carpaccio with Parmesan (p232)** Home-made bitter almond milky jelly	**Vegetable tartare with chopped smoked salmon (p174)** Spaghetti Bolognese with 40g (1½oz) Parmesan cheese Home-made chocolate-flavoured egg custard	Prawn cocktail with American sauce Duck tournedos, polenta with sun-dried tomatoes **Chocolate mousse with stem ginger and candied orange peel (p282)**
Virtually fat-free quark **Oat bran galette (p143)**	Fat-free vanilla-flavoured yoghurt **Oat bran galette (p143)**	Fat-free coconut-flavoured yoghurt	Virtually fat-free quark
Chilled cucumber and mint soup Big American salad: crab, carrots, ¼ grapefruit, prawns, celery, Maya salad dressing Home-made coffee granita with cinnamon	Tzatziki Sardines, grilled, barbecued or cooked in the oven Steamed vegetables with Dukan aïoli sauce **Extra-light strawberry mousse (p196)**	**Pissaladière slices (p213)** **Sautéed Mediterranean prawns with caramelized ginger (p146)** Roasted fennel Fresh raspberries	Tomato and pepper salad **Mushroom, bresaola and fruity Gouda slices (p233)** Rocket salad Home-made lemon mousse

Autumn Menu

	MONDAY	TUESDAY	WEDNESDAY
	Pure Proteins	**Proteins Vegetables**	**Proteins Vegetables Fruit**
Breakfast	Fat-free fromage frais Turkey breast **Oat bran galette (p143)**	Fat-free cottage cheese **Oat bran galette (p143)** Home-made rhubarb compote	Home-made egg custard 1 orange Oat bran muffin
Lunch	Prawns Lemon, lemon-grass and ginger chicken strips **Konjac shirataki noodles, (p171)** lemony fromage frais sauce Fat-free coconut-flavoured yoghurt	Chicory salad Beef burger with onions French beans Fat-free strawberry-flavoured yoghurt	Home-made chicken liver terrine Grilled turkey escalope Fried or steamed courgettes Fat-free lemon-flavoured yoghurt
Snack	Fat-free cottage cheese with cinnamon	Virtually fat-free quark	Fat-free fromage frais
Dinner	Beef carpaccio with balsamic dressing **Veal with thyme and lemon (p150)** Vanilla fromage frais mousse	Tomato, pepper and onion salad **Dukan Neapolitan pizza (p175)** Home-made egg custard, flavour of your choice	Wild mushroom velouté **Two tomato tortilla (p169)** Dukan floating islands

Autumn Menu

THURSDAY	FRIDAY	SATURDAY	SUNDAY
Proteins Vegetables Fruit Bread	**Proteins Vegetables Fruit Bread Cheese**	**Proteins Vegetables Fruit Bread Cheese Starchy Foods**	**Day with a celebration meal**
50g (1¾oz) toasted wholemeal bread Fat-free fromage frais Home-made rhubarb compote	**Oat bran galette (p143)** Fat-free cottage cheese 1 soft-boiled egg	50g (1¾oz) toasted wholemeal bread Fat-free fromage frais with cinnamon Home-made rhubarb compote	**Oat bran galette (p143)** Fat-free cottage cheese Home-made rhubarb compote
Ham or turkey fat-free quark rolls **Mountain salad with Tomme de Savoie (p234)** and bresaola Fat-free honey-flavoured yoghurt	Steamed artichoke with Maya salad dressing **Konjac tagliatelle carbonara (p173)** Brussels sprouts 40g (1½oz) Camembert cheese	Grated carrot salad Mushroom and potato omelette Mixed salad Fat-free cottage cheese	Assortment of North African starters Couscous royal Nougat glacé
Virtually fat-free quark	Fat-free coconut-flavoured yoghurt	**Oat bran galette (p143)**	Virtually fat-free quark
Mackerel fillets in white wine sauce **Moroccan-style mussels (p149)** Carrots cooked with garlic and cumin Home-made spicy custard	**Pissaladière slices (p213)** and salad Ham and chicory with Dukan béchamel sauce **Apple, pear and raspberry crumble (p195)**	**Small squash with Comté (p231)** Boiled beef and vegetable stew Mandarin and orange salad with cinnamon and orange flower water	**Porcini mushroom velouté (p168)** **Mushroom, bresaola and fruity Gouda slices (p233)** Baked apple

Girlfriends Together Menu

	MONDAY	TUESDAY	WEDNESDAY
	Pure Proteins	**Proteins Vegetables**	**Proteins Vegetables Fruit**
Breakfast	Fat-free fromage frais Turkey breast **Oat bran galette (p143)**	Fat-free fromage frais **Oat bran galette (p143)** Home-made rhubarb compote	Home-made egg custard Oat bran muffin
Lunch	Fat-free cottage cheese with chopped fresh herbs Seafood platter: prawns, mussels, marinated fish, scallops Fat-free vanilla-flavoured yoghurt	Chilled cucumber and mint soup Big Niçoise salad: French beans, tuna, tomatoes, anchovy, radish, red pepper, hard-boiled egg, Maya salad dressing Virtually fat-free quark, fig-flavoured	Gazpacho Big American salad: crab, carrots, grapefruit, prawns, celery, Maya salad dressing Fat-free strawberry-flavoured yoghurt
Snack	Fat-free fromage frais with cinnamon	Fat-free cottage cheese	Virtually fat-free quark
Dinner	Tuna soufflé Salmon fillet parcel with lime Dukan floating islands, crème anglaise with matcha green tea	Finely chopped fennel salad with lemon Seared tuna steak, cooked on one side only, basil fromage frais sauce and spinach Home-made egg custard, flavour of your choice	Smoked salmon slices Mediterranean prawn kebabs, steamed broccoli Home-made Dukan recipe egg custard

Girlfriends Together Menu

THURSDAY	FRIDAY	SATURDAY	SUNDAY
Proteins Vegetables Fruit Bread	**Proteins Vegetables Fruit Bread Cheese**	**Proteins Vegetables Fruit Bread Cheese Starchy Foods**	**Day with a celebration meal**
50g (1¾oz) toasted wholemeal bread Fat-free fromage frais Home-made rhubarb compote	50g (1¾oz) toasted wholemeal bread Fat-free cottage cheese 1 soft-boiled egg	50g (1¾oz) toasted wholemeal bread Fat-free fromage frais with cinnamon Home-made rhubarb compote	50g (1¾oz) toasted wholemeal bread Fat-free cottage cheese Egg white omelette
Vegetable smoothie: carrot, beetroot, celery Big pink and salmon salad: salmon, pink grapefruit, radish, spinach, beetroot, Maya salad dressing Dukan coconut lumps with oat bran	Coleslaw: grated carrot, cabbage and onion Dukan beef burger: minced beef, tomatoes, salad, gherkins, diet ketchup in 2 small oat bran galettes Coffee milkshake: fat-free yoghurt, skimmed milk, coffee or 1 teaspoon instant coffee, ice cubes	Lemon marinated chicken mini-kebabs **Double salmon tartare with red quinoa (p257)** and steamed vegetables Fat-free lemon-flavoured yoghurt	Toast with pâté and pine nut salad Complete raclette: potatoes, raclette cheese, bresaola **Japanese-style chocolate fondant (p281)**
Virtually fat-free quark	Fat-free coconut-flavoured yoghurt	½ **oat bran galette (p143)**	**Oat bran galette (p143)**
Japanese salad: cucumber and nori seaweed Sashimi and grated black winter radish Coconut-flavoured agar-agar jelly (or coconut-flavoured fat-free yoghurt) and lychees	Artichoke heart and lemon salad **Spinach and goat's cheese gratin (p236)** **Mint sorbet with strawberry coulis (p190)**	Cherry tomato and basil salad **Beef carpaccio with Parmesan (p232)** and rocket salad **Vanilla cheese-cake with raspberry coulis (p193)**	Raita salad with cucumber, garlic and yoghurt **Tandoori chicken with red lentil dhal (p260)** Rose water lassi ½ mango

Romantic Tête-À-Tête Menu

	MONDAY		WEDNESDAY
	Pure Proteins	**Proteins Vegetables**	**Proteins Vegetables Fruit**
Breakfast	Fat-free fromage frais Turkey breast **Oat bran galette (p143)**	Fat-free cottage cheese **Oat bran galette (p143)** Home-made rhubarb compote	Home-made egg custard Oat bran muffin Egg white omelette with freshly chopped herbs
Lunch	Fresh herb and fat-free fromage frais omelette **Veal with thyme and lemon (p150)** Konjac shirataki noodles, fromage frais lemon sauce Fat-free cottage cheese with vanilla seeds	Raita salad with cucumber, garlic and yoghurt **Tandoori chicken (p260)** and red 'ratatouille': tomatoes-courgettes-red peppers Fat-free coconut-flavoured yoghurt	Bresaola and gherkins Skirt of beef with shallots Braised chicory Fat-free coconut-flavoured yoghurt
Snack	Fat-free fromage frais with cinnamon	Fat-free cottage cheese	Virtually fat-free quark
Dinner	Dublin Bay prawns Fresh salmon fillet parcels with ginger Jasmine tea granita	Dukan recipe eggs cocotte with prawns Sea bream tartare with lemon, ginger and red berries Artichoke hearts, carrot and celeriac cooked in lemon juice Soy milk ginger agar-agar cream	Tuna and beetroot mousse Dukan crab cake Tomato, alfalfa sprouts and mixed leaf salad Fruit gratin with blueberries

Romantic Tête-À-Tête Menu

THURSDAY	FRIDAY	SATURDAY	SUNDAY
Proteins Vegetables Fruit Bread	**Proteins Vegetables Fruit Bread Cheese**	**Proteins Vegetables Fruit Bread Cheese Starchy Foods**	Day with a celebration meal
Oat bran galette (p143) Fat-free fromage frais Home-made rhubarb compote	25g(1oz) toasted wholemeal bread Fat-free cottage cheese 1 soft-boiled egg	Oat bran muffin Fat-free fromage frais with cinnamon Fresh orange and lemon juice	50g (1¾oz) toasted wholemeal bread Fat-free cottage cheese Egg white omelette
Smoked salmon slices with 50g (1¾oz) toasted wholemeal bread Cod fillet with Dukan aioli-style vegetables Home-made fruit salad	Chicory and mature Mimolette salad Roast chicken French beans Fruits of the forest syllabub	Hot goat's cheese salad **Orange and red striped salmon slices (p215)** Bed of fresh wilted spinach Home-made chocolate-flavoured egg custard	**'Assiette gourmande' (p277)** Champagne, salmon and Dublin Bay prawns sauerkraut **Chocolate mousse with stem ginger and candied orange peel (p282)**
Fat-free strawberry-flavoured yoghurt	Fat-free fromage frais Oat bran muffin	Fat-free vanilla-flavoured yoghurt	**Oat bran galette (p143)**
Courgette velouté Beef meatballs with mint and baked aubergine millefeuille Home-made spicy custard	A dozen oysters with 25g (1oz) rye or wholemeal bread Saffron mussel stew: mussels, carrots, turnips, cabbage, leeks Dukan Diet chocolate fondant	Gazpacho **Chicken liver risotto (p254)** Provençal-style tomatoes Dukan-style rhubarb clafoutis	**Carpaccio of fresh salmon and goat's cheese (p235)** Provençal-style scallops and red 'ratatouille': tomatoes-courgettes-red peppers Dukan recipe praline bavarois and slivers of pears

If, by following my programme, you've got
to this point on your road map and you've
achieved your True Weight, well done!
However, as far as your weight in the future is concerned, you
need to understand that you're now at a point of no return.

• 50 per cent of my patients stop here because they consider
themselves cured. However, they forget that there are still two
more phases to get through. And it's these two phases alone
that will ensure you stay at this weight over the long term.
All these impatient folk, without exception, will
either put the weight back on or their eating will
get so muddled that it can only end in failure.
So you've been warned.

• The other 50 per cent don't stop here; they follow me into
the third phase, Consolidation. And 85 per cent of them make
it right to the end and manage to consolidate their weight.
They're on the right track but they still
haven't completed their journey.
Only those who follow the fourth and final phase,
permanent Stabilization, and incorporate it into their
daily routine succeed in achieving the only goal that
counts – 'being cured of being overweight'.

Dear reader, I hope with all my heart that you won't
end your diet at this point and that you'll carry on with
our joint undertaking until you reach the very end. My
dearest wish is to see you succeed and win the battle.

The Consolidation Phase

You've just conquered your True Weight and it belongs to you, so the time has come to work out together what will happen to it from now on. If you follow me, I can absolutely promise you this: if you do the Consolidation phase, which is usually quite short and surprisingly easy, and then go through the permanent Stabilization phase, YOU WILL NEVER, EVER PUT ANY WEIGHT BACK ON AGAIN.

I can make you this promise with such certainty because I have a database tracking people I've been treating for over 15 years who have never regained any weight. Tens of thousands of people have achieved this goal and, when I ask these men and women about it, they all speak of their deep and genuine satisfaction – their lives have changed.

You may well be asking yourself why I'm so desperately keen to get my readers to lose weight. Quite simply because it's what I do best – it has become my life and my raison d'être. If you were one of these people who slim down and remain slimmed down, then as a doctor I'd know that I've accomplished what I set out to accomplish.

Many people put weight back on after dieting and there's a simple explanation: they aren't offered a structured, concrete and simple model to help them preserve what they've worked so hard to achieve. And this is a real shame.

This is why, as far back as 1985, I started working on finding ways to counteract the natural tendency to regain weight. Our bodies store away fat reserves; it's what they're programmed to do. Fat, whether animal or plant, is closely bound up with survival, and our genes and metabolism are completely unaware that food has become so abundant nowadays.

In my original method, the first front, I devoted two of the four phases to achieving consolidation–stabilization. If you've used other methods, you'll have noticed that once you've slimmed down, there's plenty of advice about common sense and moderation. The same advice you see on the TV adverts that remind you to eat a balanced diet, in moderation and take exercise while at the same time showing you images of caramel melting over chocolate or hamburgers containing almost 1,000 calories.

Almost everyone who has put weight back on after losing it with my method has done so because they didn't follow the Consolidation and then the Stabilization phases.

The obesity study that dealt with 4,500 women, the largest study to look at my method, showed that the women who regained weight after losing it did not follow these two crucial phases. A third of them state that they're ready to follow the diet again, but that this time they'd carry on right until the very end.

The Consolidation phase which I'm asking you to follow is a sort of decompression chamber; it's absolutely vital after any weight loss.

Whichever of my two fronts you follow – the strong way or the gentle way – they both have this phase. And I suggest that anyone finishing a diet, of any sort, even if it isn't mine, should use it because no other current diet has devised a decompression chamber like this one, acting as a transition between dieting and not dieting.

There's no shortage of diets out there, from the most far-fetched to the most extreme and even dangerous ones. However, if you're searching for proper tools to maintain yourself at your new hard-won weight, then there's a big nothing.

I know from experience both how difficult it is to lose weight in a world that encourages you to put it on, and the joy that comes from losing it. However, I'm equally aware of how miserable it is to put weight back on. So I'm campaigning to get nutritionists to realize that, so long as you make every effort to stabilize all you've accomplished, weight regain after dieting is not a foregone conclusion.

For 15 years I worked on the post-dieting period that follows on directly from significant weight loss and runs until the end of your life. It took me a great deal of time and effort to shape the Consolidation and Stabilization phases, since it's easier to establish a one-off project with a negotiated timescale – losing weight – than it is to ensure you keep to your True Weight and that it lasts over time. For me, as for you, this was the challenge I had to take up. Achieving it is far more technical and requires much greater experience, expertise and insight into the particular psychology of overweight people.

To avoid weight regain, you have to overcome what I call '**the rebound phenomenon**'. It is a natural response by the body which, in order to protect its reserves of vital energy, tries to replenish them once they run out. As soon as you start dieting, this phenomenon kicks in, gathering force as you continue your diet in a vain attempt to thwart it. Once dieting is over, it intensifies as your body tries to get back the pounds you've lost.

All these physiological actions were designed to help get us through times of famine and food shortages, when it was impossible to find enough to eat. They are meant to protect you. Nowadays they work against you, firstly by preventing you from losing weight; and secondly, when you do manage to slim down, by encouraging weight regain. To put it in a nutshell: you're living in a body that wants to stop you losing weight and in a world that's making you put it on.

If what you're aiming for is to lose weight and keep it off, it's very important that you understand what is going on inside you while you're dieting and thereafter. The real problem with being overweight is weight regain. I can't recall having met an overweight or even an obese patient who hadn't at least once in their lives managed to get down to a healthy weight.

Is the rebound phenomenon identical to what the media have named 'the yo-yo effect'? No, the yo-yo effect as such doesn't exist. This term implies that, as with an actual yo-yo toy, having gone down, your weight bounces back up to the starting point and each time goes up even higher. This argument is inaccurate and was dreamt up to discourage people who want to lose weight. Lots of studies have shown that, following weight loss, our metabolism reverts to its previous state. It is, of course, possible to put on more than was lost – not for physio-logical reasons, but for psychological ones. So anyone suffering from stress and experiencing dissatisfaction in their lives would carry on gaining weight whether they were dieting or not.

On the other hand, it's clear that whatever the diet, or whatever the cause of the weight loss, this tendency towards regain is systematic, simply because it's normal.

Please note, I said *tendency* and not regain.

According to my statistics, half of my readers, with the help solely of a road map from a book, have kept all the weight off one year after finishing the diet.

And 25 per cent have maintained their True Weight after five years.

With daily, interactive internet coaching, the percent-age goes up to almost 70 per cent after one year and to 35 per cent after five years.

Controlling Rebound

You've just attained your True Weight. All the time you were shedding weight, your body tried to react and stop this happening. You may have noticed this each time you went through the week and came to Friday. However, each week the first four days forced your body to let go of a little of your surplus weight.

Today, you're shifting gear. Together we're going to widen your diet. The reactions your body has unsuccessfully put in place are now gathering force to make you regain the weight you've just lost. It's really worth your while understanding this, so you can foil its attempts.

In both the animal and the plant kingdom, storing calories away as fat reserves is a fundamental function. Olive oil or fat in a hedgehog serve the same purpose, play the same role: they allow the plant or animal to survive. It's just the same for humans, and anyone who takes in more energy than their body expends will keep the surplus in reserve. Nature or evolution 'invented' fat reserves as the material and biological nutrient capable of concentrating the most energy in the smallest volume (1g of fat = 9 calories). A person can live for almost a week from just one kilo of fat. For our ancestors surviving in hostile environments, whose food supply fluctuated according to the seasons and animal migrations, this was useful and protected them. What's more, throughout the 190,000 years of primitive life, then during the periods of famine that have recurred during our history, evolution has selected those bodies with the thriftiest metabolism.

If you want to get your mind around weight problems, you need to take on board this simple, but crucial fact: your body, such as it is now, was designed not only to adapt and survive in an environment where subsistence was hard, but also to be far more physically active than is necessary today.

This amounts to saying that our bodies, metabolisms, instincts and behaviour patterns have remained unchanged since the Paleolithic Age. We may not have altered, but over the past 60 years or so the world we've been living in has undergone profound change. What was useful in the past – storing fat – is completely unnecessary and works against you. If you want to learn what to do to avoid putting back on the pounds you've lost, it's vital that you bear this in mind.

How does your body try to resist weight loss and get you to store fat away again? I've listed three ways:

1. The first is to trigger and stimulate a sensation of hunger, creating a behaviour pattern that gives you a strong appetite for food. The more frustrating the diet has been and the longer it has gone on, the more powerful this reaction will be.

2. The body's second way is to cut down on the energy it uses. When a person has a drop in salary, their first reaction is to reduce any outgoings. The body does likewise. This explains why many patients on a weight-loss diet complain about feeling cold; the body is using less energy

to keep itself warm. The same thing is happening if you feel tired; the body is trying to curb unnecessary physical effort. Any excessive activity becomes burdensome. This is why, for the first three days of the week in particular, I advised you to simply go for a walk. It's the only exercise that doesn't tire you out or make you feel hungry.

3. Finally, the body's third reaction – and the most unwelcome for anyone trying to stabilize at their new weight – is to extract the maximum from any food consumed. So someone who'd normally extract 100 calories from a harmless bread roll manages the feat of extracting 120–130 when dieting.

To do this, the body sifts through each foodstuff until it gives up its 'very substance'. This high-performance calorie extraction takes place in the small intestine, the interface between the bloodstream and the rest of the body. Moreover, this is where oat bran comes into its own, by slowing down the assimilation of calories and by taking a few of them away into the stools. You can see why it's so important.

INCREASE IN APPETITE + REDUCTION IN ENERGY USED + MAXIMUM CALORIE EXTRACTION = YOU BECOME A PROPER CALORIE SPONGE!

And, generally it's at this point that some dieters, satisfied with their results, think they can now go easy. They fall back into their old ways and this is the most natural and common reason for quickly regaining weight.

This means that the risk of regain is at its greatest immediately after successful dieting, when the target weight has been reached. This is the so-called rebound period because, like a ball that has just touched the ground, weight naturally tends to rebound. And it's during this ultra-vulnerable period that ALL current diets stop offering any proper, structured, easy-to-follow instructions that set boundaries. Instead, they give you some pitiful advice about using common sense. This allows your body to do what it likes and follow the rigid determinism of its automatic responses.

If you're delighted at having got back your body, your image, your health and beauty, if your life has changed and you're satisfied with it, be aware that this will all melt away like butter left in the sun if you fail to heed the programmes for Consolidation and for Stabilization.

How Long Will This Rebound Reaction Last?

Once I decided to work on this post-diet period, I searched around in previous works to find estimates for the length of time this rebound phase lasts, which so often causes immediate failure. I couldn't find any precise timing, only confirmation that the rebound would gradually peter out and the body would revert to its initial metabolic status. As with smokers who've weaned themselves off tobacco, withdrawal stops slowly but surely. So it's important to know how long the rebound will last so that, within this set time frame, you can fight it with an appropriate strategy and defensive diet.

I decided therefore to work out the length of time by monitoring what happened to a large number of my patients once they'd lost weight. This allowed me to define the vulnerability to weight regain.

Based on my observations, I concluded that **the time you remain vulnerable depends on how much weight you've lost and lasts approximately five days for every pound lost**, i.e. around 30 days or a month for 6 pounds, 100 days for 20 pounds.

For you this is both good and bad news:

- The bad news is that after losing weight, you'll be prone to a natural tendency to put back the weight you've lost. Knowing this, you can take steps to protect yourself and I'm going to help you.
- The good news is that this period is time-limited, so you'll know precisely how long it will last.

Armed with this knowledge, you're alerted to the danger and for how long. This should get you to accept, without too much difficulty, the extra work required to neutralize the rebound.

Reactive, cautious and on the alert, your body will calm down, simply with the passing of time, provided you don't overindulge. Eventually it will stop wanting to retrieve the weight you've lost. A calm sea is awaiting you at the end of the tunnel, I promise you.

Then my permanent Stabilization programme, with its three simple, concrete and pain-free measures, including the famous Protein Thursdays, will complete your journey over the long term.

To get through this risky but well-defined period, where so many people come unstuck, I've constructed the Consolidation phase.

The instructions that will guide you are sufficiently precise, simple, concrete and rewarding to ward off the threat of rebound until it dies away. This new programme isn't a diet but a channel that will steer you to your destination. Your eating will remain on track, you'll be free to eat so that you stop losing weight but you'll still be protected by a certain number of guidelines that will prevent you from putting any back on.

True Weight's Major Role

As the Persian proverb says, 'There is no fair wind for those who know not to where they sail.'

The same is true for anyone who first wants to lose weight but in particular stabilize it afterwards – they have to know the weight they're aiming for.

What is this weight? In many countries, and this has been going on for ages, women have felt cultural pressure to be slim, extremely slim even. Men have ended up feeling this cultural pressure, too. However, reason has to prevail. I've witnessed too many failures that were mainly down to setting unrealistic target weights.

For any attempt to slim to be successful and lasting, it's important that the target weight is both 'attainable' and 'maintainable'. Many weights are attainable but that doesn't mean they're all maintainable.

If you've already tried losing weight, you'll know that there are weight zones that you can attain relatively easily, others that are more difficult and lastly extreme zones to which, whatever diet you try, your weight will never drop down. Normally it's in these zones that you experience the 'stagnation plateau' challenge. Despite following your diet correctly, your weight won't shift. There's no point in trying to stabilize your weight in this zone, because the effort required to attain it – already disproportionate at the outset – and then to maintain it afterwards would demand such heroism that you wouldn't be able to sustain it over the long term.

So it's totally inappropriate to set a stabilization weight that doesn't suit your nature. What you need is to be able to live normally, and go for a weight with which you feel comfortable. Lastly, you need to take into account the maximum and minimum weight you've ever reached. Because no matter how long you stayed at this maximum weight, it's forever etched into your body – your body has its memory. Let's take an example: imagine a woman about 5 feet 6 inches tall who, on a single day of her life, weighed around 15½ stone. It's absolutely impossible for this woman to ever hope to stabilize at around 8 stone, as some theoretical tables suggest she could. It's just not realistic.

However, suggesting to her that she attains and maintains her weight at around 11 stone on paper seems far wiser, provided of course that she feels comfortable at this weight.

Finally, you need to dispel another common misconception. Most of you imagine that you'll stabilize better at a certain weight if you slim down a little more, so that you've got a couple of pounds or so as a safety margin to give you some leeway if you have to react. For example, wanting to slim down to 10 stone something so that you stabilize at around 11 isn't just wrong, it's a huge mistake because you'd be wasting the willpower you'll need come the time to start stabilizing at your chosen weight.

And, most importantly – the more you try to get your weight down, the more your body will react and there'll be a greater tendency to rebound upwards! Always bear this in mind.

So to succeed in this difficult task of curing yourself of being overweight, you have to choose a weight that you can both attain AND stabilize, i.e. a weight that's high enough for you to achieve without getting lost on the way, but low enough for you to feel great, rewarded, and encouraged to maintain and protect it.

True Weight is what I've called this weight.

How Is True Weight Determined and Worked Out?

First of all, you are no doubt aware of the standard international weight index, used more or less worldwide, called the Body Mass Index, or BMI. All health professionals employ this tool, and it's very handy for identifying high-risk populations. However, BMI is less useful for determining an individual's weight because only two parameters, weight and height, are used to calculate it. The BMI wasn't enough for me when I was working with my patients. It didn't take gender into consideration, which is so important for weight, or age, or a person's weight background with its fluctuations, or the number of pregnancies, or skeleton size.

Nonetheless, like a lot of doctors, I used it for want of anything better. And often I had to deal with patients who couldn't get their heads around their BMI, as it just didn't speak to them.

Over time, I made it my practice to determine weight based on what I knew about my patient. Each patient is a special case. I still remember one particular female patient who was aiming for a certain weight which, given all her attributes, was in my opinion far too low. I tried reasoning with her, explaining that she would be sacrificing some of her femininity, and she retorted amiably: 'Like all Mediterranean men, you prefer women with curves!'

She said it as a joke, but to avoid all subjectivity in assessing my patients, I developed a scientific tool for my calculations, True Weight, which includes all the relevant parameters with the respective value I allocate to each one. To do this, I had to work with a computer scientist, so that the complex calculations can be processed by an algorithm that is sufficiently sophisticated to incorporate all these parameters, yet sufficiently simple for anyone to calculate their True Weight in a few seconds.

I made sure it was ready for my coaching website so that everyone can start off their treatment by working out what their target weight should be.

How do you determine your True Weight?
By definition, this weight is personal. To be relevant and workable, it has to take into account all the elements that explain your current weight and which constitute for you, and you alone, the strategic weight that you stand the best chance of attaining and maintaining. These elements are:

- **Your current weight**, what you weigh when you're calculating it.
- **Your height** in centimetres.
- **Your gender**. A man weighs more than a woman of the same height because of muscle mass and our culture for being thin.
- **Your age**. From the age of 18, statistically a healthy weight will naturally increase with each decade by 800g (about 1¾ pounds) for women and by 1.2 kilos (over 2½ pounds) for men. If an 18-year-old girl weighs 52 kilos, she'll have to accept that at 28 she'll weigh 52.8 kilos, and 53.6 kilos at 38 and so on until she's 58.
- **The maximum weight** you've ever reached in your life (for women this doesn't include pregnancies).
- **The minimum weight** you've been, excluding all illnesses. The difference between these two weights, recorded in your body's biological memory, is what I

call 'weight range'. The wider the range, the more this will push up your True Weight. A woman whose lowest weight was just over 9 stone but who has also weighed 15½ stone will have to abandon any idea of getting back down to 9 stone.

- **The weight you've stayed at for longest**. This is a benchmark weight, a weight with which your body feels relatively at ease and which should therefore be included.
- **Family background**. If your mother or father is over-weight, this will force me to increase your True Weight, as family background plays an important role in some very specific cases, but far less of one if it's just a tendency.
- **The number of diets you've tried**. If you have a chequered dieting past, your True Weight has to take this into account. However, not all diets affect the psyche and the body's responsiveness in the same way. The ones that have the greatest impact on the body's memory are the ones furthest removed from our natural diet. This holds true for meal replacement sachets or powders because we're not programmed to live off powders. We can do it for a very short time, but eating food that is so artificial engenders such frustration that unfortunately this makes us resistant to other natural methods. Fasting, which amounts to swallowing nothing other than water, is disastrous for our muscle mass, as the body resorts to using up proteins that are vital for its survival. However, fasting is far, far more

natural than eating powders; indeed, it's quite common for a predator to be forced to fast for several days if there's no prey to be had.

· **Bone structure**. If you have a heavy bone structure, this will play a part in calculating your weight. To work it out, grasp you left wrist between your right thumb and forefinger. If both ends touch, your bone structure is normal and doesn't play any part in the calculation. If they don't touch and there's a space between them, your bone structure is heavy, and if they overlap, it's light. In both cases, your True Weight will be adjusted up or down.

· **Number of pregnancies** (for women). Each pregnancy adds almost a couple of pounds to your True Weight, but this extra amount will vary according to the number and your age.

As you can see, many parameters are involved in working out your True Weight, and they have to be included in order to determine your instructions. You'll find a free questionnaire with these 11 questions at **www.regimedu-kan.com**. If you fill out the questionnaire, you'll get your True Weight straightaway. Then you'll know exactly where to aim for your bull's-eye, you'll know the distance, and I'll give you the bow and arrow – that way you'll stand the best chance of scoring a hit.

A Practical Guide to the Consolidation Phase

Good news – if you've just finished your Nutritional Staircase phase, without even realizing it you've already started working on the Consolidation phase!

This is one of the fundamental differences with the first front.

Remember: the first front has four phases, and weight loss is achieved with high-protein foods only during the Attack phase, then proteins and vegetables during the Cruise phase until you reach your target weight.

In the second front, which is what interests you here, both major categories are only used on Monday, the day for proteins, and on Tuesday, when vegetables are added.

And from Wednesday onwards, day after day, you eat Consolidation foods. However, since you don't get them all at once, you continue losing weight until Thursday evening, then Friday and Saturday you remain in balance, and on Sunday you allow your body to breathe and replenish itself.

Now that you're starting the Consolidation phase, things will be organized differently and this is what I'm going to explain to you.

Let me remind you that to consolidate the weight you've attained, what this phase chiefly aims to do is ward off your most immediate threat – the body's natural rebound. You'll be at risk until the body's physiological reactions have calmed down, just like a wall that is solid only once the cement has set and has completely dried out.

These defence reactions are proportionate to the amount of weight lost and will go on for longer the greater the risk.

As I've explained to you, Consolidation lasts five days for each pound you've lost; it's easy and simple to calculate. Once you've worked it out, split the number of days in two so that this phase divides into two equal halves.

For example, if you've lost 20 pounds, Consolidation will last 100 days and will consist of two halves each lasting 50 days.

The First Half of Consolidation

You'll find all the Nutritional Staircase foods here. No longer in a weekly sequence, but grouped together according to the rules below.

I'll remind you of them so that you distinguish carefully between the two stages of Consolidation:

High-protein foods

These are the foods that are on the first step of the Staircase, on Monday's step.

- lean meat – the leaner cuts of beef, veal
- offal and game
- fish, all without any exception
- seafood, all without any exception

- poultry without the skin, except for flat-beaked birds (duck and goose)
- eggs
- plant proteins: tofu, seitan and tempeh
- low-fat cooked ham, chicken and turkey, bresaola
- fat-free dairy products: yoghurts, fromage frais, quark, cottage cheese

Green vegetables and uncooked vegetables
All the ones you introduced on Tuesday, when you stepped on to the second step of the Staircase. The choice is immense.

During the weight-loss period, I asked you to eat them as freely as you wanted, but without forcing yourself. Given how open and diverse the seven steps were, your priority was to avoid getting dangerously bogged down in weight stagnation. Now, with quite a different situation, we're aiming to avoid any weight regain during the weeks in Consolidation.

SO THE INSTRUCTION FOR VEGETABLES IS NO LONGER 'AS MUCH AS YOU WANT' BUT 'AS MUCH AS YOU CAN'.

From now on, and for the rest of your life, a competition will be played out for foods to fill up your stomach, the organ for digestion and satiety. As I've told you, whatever your weight problem background, a stomach has its limits.

You've got to disregard the common misconception that your stomach expands as you grow overweight and obese. It's not your stomach that adapts; it's your *brain* that's always asking for more! It's very important that you understand this. What's more, in such situations, as the stomach distends it creates discomfort to which your brain also grows accustomed. So as soon as the stomach's contents reach the duodenum and small intestine, it reverts back to its initial size. This means your stomach's capacity has physical limits, which vary depending on your size and genes, but it very seldom exceeds 2.5 litres (4½ pints).

Strategically this is a very important fact: filling up your stomach needs to take into account the law of 'first come, first absorbed'. **As many vegetables as possible** means that any mouthful of greens you absorb will de facto take the place of another food. Apart from water and konjac, no food is totally devoid of calories, yet there's no other known food as rich in vitamins, mineral salts and antioxidants for so few calories as vegetables, and therefore they're great for filling up your stomach. Some bariatric surgeons employ a similar strategy when they insert a gastric balloon inside the stomach of obese patients to limit the amount they eat. Personally, I prefer vegetables!

Do remember, though, that certain vegetables, such as carrots and beetroot, contain more carbs than others. So I'd advise you to go easy on them, especially if you or any relatives are prone to diabetes.

One piece of fruit a day
Fruit was on the third step of the Staircase, on Wednesday's step.

Be wary of fruit – it contains fast carbs. Eat too much and you'll create fat to store away. Remember how insulin makes it easy to store sugar as fat. Remember, too, what I told you about fruit in the hunter-gatherer's diet, and the role it played.

Thereafter, as farming appeared and developed, fruit was selected and modified to have more and more sugar, more and more flavour, but less and less fibre. Nowadays, fruit is imported from all over the world.

So be careful when you're eating fruit. And avoid eating fruit as juice.

In the second half of Consolidation, you'll be allowed to have a second piece of fruit a day. Once you exceed this dose, fruit plays no useful nutritional role. Your vitamin and antioxidant requirements have already been met. Each additional piece of fruit only provides sugar. If you want to boost your antioxidant intake, bear in mind that vegetables are 'sugar-free fruits' and that, along with proteins, they're your best food friends.

Two slices of wholegrain or wholemeal bread
These are the two slices of bread that appeared on Thursday, on the fourth step of the Nutritional Staircase. Bread made from white flour and bread made with wholegrain flour are worlds apart. Wholegrain flour contains the antidote to violent sugar and white flour. I

know that doing without that mythical loaf of bread may prove somewhat difficult; you'll be up in arms along with all the bakers who'll be cursing me! Christianity has turned bread into something sacred; and our proverbs show how much we regard it as a vital food. However, if eaten in large amounts, white bread is nowadays a high-risk and even a dangerous food. Most bakers also produce excellent wholegrain bread, as well as a range of cereal breads that had been forgotten about but which are very tasty indeed. Nibbling on a loaf of white bread isn't just a harmless weakness. It's a way of shortening your life, making diabetes considerably worse or helping a cancer spread that has already been diagnosed.

STARTING TODAY, MAKE THIS INSTRUCTION PART OF YOUR WAY OF EATING FROM NOW ON: 'WHOLEGRAIN BREAD, YES. WHITE BREAD, I'LL AVOID AS MUCH AS POSSIBLE.'

It's increasingly common for top restaurants to offer their guests a choice of different brown bread rolls. This should be more widespread. Wholemeal bread, low-fat dairy products and cheeses, all nicely presented, certainly wouldn't discourage any customers.

And don't forget that most processed wholemeal bread is just white bread disguised by the addition of wheat bran and it's just as fat-producing (lipogenic) as white bread. Check the labels carefully, and if there's nothing suitable always go for wholegrain instead.

40g (1½oz) cheese

This is the portion you found on Friday, on the fifth step of the Nutritional Staircase. From now on, you're allowed cheese every day. However, bear in mind that once the fat content exceeds 50% we're no longer looking at a simple cheese but at a fat, and it wouldn't make sense for it to be included in your Consolidation phase – when you want to avoid producing any fat. Over 40% fat, cheese is a food for pleasure, especially because of the creamy texture.

Let me remind you about Tomme de Savoie, a cheese that deserves to be more widely known. Of all the cheeses produced in France, of all our 'appellations contrôlées', Tomme is by far the best placed to be part of a programme tackling weight and obesity. Its main advantage is that it's made from semi-skimmed milk. The traditional 12% fat recipe is a pure marvel. I've been enjoying it for over 30 years and really miss it whenever I'm abroad!

One portion of starchy foods a week

This is what awaited you on the sixth step of the Nutritional Staircase, Saturday's step. In the first half of Consolidation, you're allowed starchy foods once a week; and in the second half, twice a week.

Starchy foods make up a very large food category, a disparate group far removed from the original starch. This means that all these starchy foods pose different threats to your weight. Once again, it's not about the number of calories, but about invasiveness, texture, how quickly they get into the bloodstream, get assimilated and digested, and how quickly they raise your blood sugar level. Bearing all this in mind, it's important to choose and prepare them carefully. To sum up, you're allowed:

- 210g (7½oz) lentils, beans and chickpeas
- 200g (7oz) quinoa
- 190g (6½oz) cooked al dente pasta
- 190g (6½oz) grilled corn on the cob
- 170g (6oz) well-cooked pasta
- 170g (6oz) brown rice
- 160g (5¾oz) tinned sweetcorn
- 150g (5½oz) white rice
- 140g (5oz) baked potato
- 80g (3oz) mashed potato

For further explanations about starchy foods, refer back to my advice for Saturday.

One celebration meal a week
This is what you got used to having every Sunday on the final step of the Nutritional Staircase. From now on, you don't have to keep it for Sundays; you're free to choose the day and the occasion to enjoy it. And some good news: in the second half of the Consolidation phase, not one but two celebration meals await you! Make these meals an enjoyable time that you spend with family or friends. Get accustomed to differentiating between food that's there to provide nutrition and other food that offers pleasure and freedom. And, in the case of the latter, linger

on every mouthful and savour the effects. When you love, you're in no hurry to see the signs of love disappear!

Thursday, a pure protein day that stands guard
This day is devoted to high-protein foods. You're well acquainted with it since you started the week with pure proteins on the first step of the Nutritional Staircase. This day is an extra way of guaranteeing that your True Weight gets properly consolidated. It acts as a buffer that protects the six other days of the week, evening out any problems. Please note: Protein Thursday is not optional; it's part of this phase's overall equation. I designed it with its highs and lows, so that as a whole it would allow you to maintain your True Weight for a long enough period while it's still vulnerable, without putting any weight back on.

Lean meat, fish and seafood, poultry, eggs, low-fat sliced cooked meats, dairy products and tofu – everything, without any restriction on quantity, timing or combination. Ring the changes; try to select from the list of foods those you enjoy most and, on this day in particular, make time to cook so that you don't grow bored.

Drink plenty and, when you wake up the next morning, weigh yourself and see how well your Protein Thursday worked. This way you'll convince yourself to always keep to it.

The Second Half of Consolidation

This second half is the logical continuation of the first. By this point you've already managed to maintain your weight long enough for your body's physiological tendency to revert to its initial weight to have partly calmed down. As the spring has been released, I can now make a certain number of additions to your diet. These additions are principally carb foods and you know just how very dangerous they are. However, I believe that your body is now ready to accept them.

- The first addition is a **second piece of fruit a day**.
- The second is **the second portion of starchy foods a week**.
- The third is the **second celebration meal**.

To avoid any error in interpretation, here's a summary of the two halves of the Consolidation phase:

The first half of Consolidation
All the permitted protein foods
All vegetables
One piece of fruit a day
Two slices of wholemeal bread
One 40g (1½oz) portion of mature cheese
One portion of starchy foods a week
One celebration meal a week
Second half of Consolidation
All the permitted protein foods
All vegetables
TWO pieces of fruit a day
Two slices of wholemeal bread

One 40g (1½oz) portion of mature cheese
TWO portions of starchy foods a week
TWO celebration meals a week

ONE PIECE OF ADVICE YOU MUST KEEP

Follow the second half of this phase to the letter; you can have everything that's there. However, be careful: you're working at the margins and you really mustn't allow yourself anything extra, especially during the first weeks. Remember that time is on your side: with each week that passes, your body will come to realize that the ordeal is over, but also that your diet is filling out and slowly reverting to normal. What this phase helps you to do is evaluate through practice how important the food groups are respectively. This develops good habits that ingrain a preference for foods that are healthy and good, and make you wary and cautious of foods that can make you fat, the very foods that put your health at risk.

Today, your diet has opened out to such an extent that it very largely meets all your requirements. You have the energy you need to live and to live well, but without any possibility of producing reserves, i.e. without getting fat again. With this diet, you're getting all the nutrients you need, all the vitamins, mineral salts and fibre. **You do not lack anything**.

As a doctor and nutritionist, I'd add that you could live the rest of your life following this diet. If you managed to do this, you'd certainly live not only a longer life but, most importantly, a healthier one.

Over the last few decades, since 1970, life expectancy has increased markedly, but our quality of life during these additional 20 or so years will be very dependent on our state of health. For anyone who can live through these years without repercussions from cardiac disease or strokes, without excessive diabetes, without cancer but also with 'all their marbles', this extra quarter portion of life will be an incredible gift.

However, for anyone who isn't quite so lucky, it will be a poisoned chalice and seem more like a punishment.

So you could live your whole life and be healthy by keeping your diet in line with the second half of Consolidation, with its two pieces of fruit a day, its two portions of starchy foods and its two celebration meals a week.

Our ancestors would have been more than happy with this dietary programme. But we can't stop here, because over the past 50 years so many other foods have appeared on the scene. They're here with us, you've tasted them and your body remembers all those wonderfully gratifying carbs and fats; we can't just ignore them. I've taken them into account by creating the following Stabilization phase, so that it can be fully part of our modern life and world – part of our 'air-conditioned hell', which Arthur Miller referred to when he railed against the artificiality of the American consumerist dream, the brutality in society and the loss of human values.

The Force of Necessity

When I was a child and up to the age of 18, I lived on the fourth floor of a block of flats, which had no lift. I used to run up the stairs quite happily without giving it a second thought. And until the end of his life, my grandfather did the same. I now live in a block of flats that has a lift, yet I still walk up the stairs. I got into the habit of telling my patients not to take the lift, but I'd be lying if I told you that this lovely lift doesn't tempt me. **There's a world of difference between doing without a temptation that doesn't exist and refusing to be tempted by one that does exist**. The strength and magic of a diet that lasts the distance is that it creates strong enough guidance and structure to come close to creating conditions of necessity.

This virtual necessity is based on a structure, an amalgamation of rituals, a need for emulation and challenges to be met. Once you've finished the second half of the Consolidation phase, you're likely to find that you'll miss the guidance.

Don't be afraid; I'll be there to support you during 'the rest of your life after your victorious diet'. I'm aware of all the dangers, so I've prepared a framework for you, which is practically invisible but very effective, and which will offer you long-term protection.

The Stabilization Phase

If you've followed me right up to the edge of this final phase after going through the Nutritional Staircase phase and its two-part Consolidation, you should know that I'm very happy for you and proud of having brought you this far. Persuading you to give up the comfort you got from the foods that were causing your weight problems was a gamble, because your old eating habits reassured you and kept you in a certain psychological balance.

Let's just pause for a moment to look at what has been happening. If you put on weight, it's because you were bound to have been eating more than your biological and nutritional requirements. You were well aware of this, but you couldn't stop yourself. Then, one day, you decided to do something about it and this decision arose from reasons connected more often than not with your feelings and emotions. You chose to stop seeking comfort from food and switch to doing the exact opposite: controlling and being in control of your nutrition. Making this change was neither easy nor simple, so many congratulations on achieving it! I expected nothing less of you, and you've made me very happy.

After weeks of the Nutritional Staircase, you attained your True Weight. Then you devoted five days for every pound lost to consolidating your new weight by working through the two halves of the Consolidation phase. If everything has worked well, your body should be starting to get used to it.

So what could you possibly be missing today?

Nothing, apart from being free, completely and utterly free!

And that, precisely, is where the problem lies.

Up until now, between you and temptation (and the danger of succumbing to it amid chaos and confusion) stood me and the implicit pact we had agreed. You had entrusted me with this privilege and I had offered you my help and experience.

Now we've reached a crossroads, and I ask you to read and hear what I'm going to say very carefully.

If I was to leave you now with some simple recommendations and the same old advice about common sense and willpower, you'd be lost. I can assure you that you'd put your weight back on. You'd be like a tiny boat that hasn't been properly moored and gradually goes adrift, carried away by dangerous currents and tossed from side to side by unfavourable winds.

However, the time when you're supported and guided can't last forever either.

At this precise moment in the programme, if our dialogue were to stop now, your chances of keeping the weight off would be slim. This is shown by international statistics for all traditional diets, based on points or calorie-counting: five years after their diet only 3 per cent of users are still stabilized.

However, if you've succeeded with your Consolidation phase, thankfully you've lessened the danger. You've already negotiated the high-risk rebound period, the phase when many people regain weight. What's more, over an adequate period of time, your flesh has learnt the importance of healthy foods in your daily life. From now on they'll be a safety platform for you, which you can return to whenever there's any peril. I can guarantee you that they'll always be there somewhere and have something useful to offer you.

What you've learnt and the habits you've acquired during your Nutritional Staircase and the Consolidation phases significantly increase your chances of stabilizing your weight: they go up from 3 per cent to 10 per cent, or 15 per cent if you're not encumbered by any negative family history or by having tried too many unsuccessful diets.

NOW, IF YOU CONTINUE AND FOLLOW ME INTO THIS FINAL STABILIZATION PHASE, I PROMISE YOU TOTAL SUCCESS: A 100 PER CENT CHANCE OF REMAINING AT THIS WEIGHT FOR THE REST OF YOUR LIFE.

I can tell you're surprised and a little suspicious. You hear from all sides that stabilizing weight after dieting is impossible. Yes – and I'm well placed to know it – the risk is very real, great even, **but it is possible to eliminate it**

entirely. The best proof is that thousands of people have managed it. They're not Martians or robots, but ordinary people like you and me. They, too, have experienced weight regain after a diet. But they persevered and afterwards it never went back on again.

How Did They Do It?

They knew what they wanted; they'd decided this before they got started.

After losing weight and consolidating it, and finding themselves in the situation where you find yourself today, they committed to permanent stabilization with the same mindset as when they started their diet. They agreed to follow a strategic approach that got them to keep weight off for good.

And they were aware that they would have to hold to their initial conviction during the Stabilization phase.

This conviction came with a cost, but they knew that the reward made it worthwhile.

To avoid putting weight back on, to never, ever put weight on again, you simply have to do what they did: take ownership of this decision, make it part of your life plan and make it meaningful for you. And never take your current victory over your weight for granted, as if it were set in stone.

Keeping weight off after losing it is a mindset, achieved by being quietly vigilant and sticking to some acceptable restrictions in order to preserve the immense advantage of enjoying the well-being you're feeling today. And by doing this, you avoid the misery you'd feel if you failed and your weight went back on.

What you gain:

Your well-being: being able to move your body more freely, you feel lighter, find it easier to be physically active and have more stamina; you'll sleep better and enjoy a better sex life.

Your health: avoiding the risk of heart diseases, heart attack and strokes, diabetes, high blood pressure, cancer related to being overweight and Alzheimer's disease.

Your beauty: your inner image, your attractiveness, your physical presence, whether you're a male or a female reader.

Your normality: no longer feeling marginalized and no more discrimination.

Your self-confidence and your self-esteem: your pride in having been able to bring your body and body image under control. Your self-fulfilment, your quality of life, your happiness and your destiny are at stake.

These five beneficial effects are precious; they colour the quality of our lives. Important, essential and crucial, they are hard-won, but I can assure you that if you acknowledge the issues and challenges, you can succeed. You'll tell me that a 100 per cent chance for everyone is a Utopian goal, a presumptuous one even, since it doesn't allow for the ups and downs people experience in their lives. But for you, a unique individual who by losing weight has mostly got your life back under control again, it is entirely possible.

How Will You Do It?

It's no longer about keeping you safe over a limited period, using structured support, but about protecting you for the rest of your life. The Stabilization programme I'm going to suggest to you is neither off-putting nor difficult; it's feasible and sustainable, I've seen to that.

Up until now, you've been gripped by a challenge that allowed you little scope for improvisation. From now on, you'll get back your independence and the risks that come with it, which you and I know inside out. So I've marked out your new path with instructions that are simple, concrete and pain-free enough for you to be able to integrate them into your way of life easily and without feeling any frustration.

You have to keep in mind the diet you have at the first level of the Consolidation phase and combine it with three Stabilization measures.

The Safety Platform

This is the basis of your permanent stabilization. You know this food platform well: you used it all the weeks you spent on the Nutritional Staircase. And you used it in both parts of the Consolidation phase.

It is comprised of foods that meet all our human requirements. What's more, these foods are among the most natural and universal foods there are. As for the two portions of starchy foods, your daily cheese allowance and two celebration meals a week, they're far from being indispensable as far as nutrition is concerned, but they may be as regards pleasure. A portion of Reblochon, some pesto pasta or Cantonese-style rice would be your bit of luxury, your pleasure permit. Moreover, you can eat whatever vegetables, fruits, meat, fish, seafood, poultry and dairy products you want.

What's missing then from all that? Today you're bound to answer: nothing. But what about tomorrow? Because the day will come when whatever it was that made you fat comes knocking at your door again. Negative emotions such as stress, dissatisfaction, setbacks, frustrations, a break-up or bereavement, boredom, loneliness – in a nutshell, whenever you feel miserable.

If you put on weight, it was because you used food to compensate. Who is able to distance themselves from the aggression out there in the world, from a difficult social environment, from toxic consumerism? Who doesn't have tough situations to deal with in their life? How should we react in painful and tough moments?

Life comes with its challenges, but you now know how to face them without taking refuge in food. You know that there are other sources of satisfaction, there's quite a wide range to choose from. However, if you're still the same person who put that weight on at the start, if the victory you've just experienced has taught you nothing, then, yes, you will put weight back on. However, I doubt it and to tell you the truth I'm even quite sure that you've taken on board my programme, which is deliberately very structured, effective and didactic. I'm certain that you've learnt good habits and acquired sound, concrete knowledge about nutrition; enough, in any case, to feed yourself without running any risks while still enjoying lots of tasty recipes. You can't have failed to open your eyes to the reasons why you put on weight, or to the ways of neutralizing and even reversing them.

First of all, I ask you to become fully conversant with this safety platform; it has to become the basis for what you eat in the future. You'll need to make this basis a sanctuary; I value it as mankind's food heritage. From this basis everything else will become available. You can go back to eating what you want, but it's crucial that this platform becomes a safe place to which you can withdraw whenever danger looms on the horizon.

The Three Stabilization Measures

Given that I'm offering you these measures so that you integrate them into your way of life permanently, I've endeavoured to make them simple, concrete, extremely effective but also as unrestricting as possible.

Don't play around with them, they are not negotiable.

However, if you follow them regularly, I can assure you that you'll stabilize your weight, and that quite simply you'll be 'cured'. You'll do what a great number of my permanently stabilized patients and readers have done. But if you give up on them, because some problem or difficulty in life makes you vulnerable, you'll risk putting some or all of the weight you've lost back on again. So you've been warned – I know from experience!

I'm asking you to maintain a link between us, which is these three measures. This means you'll be completely autonomous, but with a safety net.

Protein Thursdays

One day a week, Thursday, will be your sentinel day, standing guard over your stability. On your Nutritional Staircase it was Monday, it was your weight-loss period and you kept to it during the Consolidation phase.

This Thursday is vital for protecting the rest of your week. It guarantees safety and gives you some leeway to eat flexibly and spontaneously over the six other days of the week. Look upon it as your insurance policy.

Many people never miss it because they've got into the habit. Protein Thursday is a part of their lives and they look forward to it because they've learnt just how useful it is. They know its power to put things right and they realize how much they owe it.

I'd like you to know the reasons why I introduced this day.

The first of these reasons is that a day of proteins, in isolation in a week when you eat freely, is, after fasting, the most powerful dietary tool available.

I often meet people at conferences or when I'm socializing who are distraught about being really overweight; they believe it's dangerous and don't feel good about themselves. They'd like to lose weight but can't make up their minds. The need is there, realization of the need to act too, but words don't translate into action; there's nothing driving it. So, often I suggest the following to them:

'Tomorrow morning, weigh yourself before you eat, and during the day eat what you want of meat, fish, seafood, poultry without the skin, low-fat cooked meats and dairy products and tofu. Drink two litres of water and walk for 30 minutes. The next morning, weigh yourself in just the same way and call me or write to me.'

The overwhelming majority of these people don't hesitate. They follow my advice and without fail they lose weight. This varies depending on how overweight they are, but it's always 2–4 pounds. And, very often, that's all it takes to make them decide to lose weight once and for all. Reason and good, logical arguments weren't enough to make up their minds; they needed something to drive them on and a day of proteins is a powerful way of boosting motivation.

In the permanent Stabilization phase, your Protein Thursday is capable all on its own of eliminating the 'little food extras' that crop up over the six other days of the week. I write 'little extras', because a Protein Thursday, as powerful and effective as it is, obviously can't mop up any bingeing that's excessive or too frequent.

The second reason for having this Protein Thursday is its value as a ritual. Humans are very susceptible to this mental phenomenon, which is similar to developing habits, and, like habits, it plays a decisive role in protecting our lives. If you've followed your Thursday two or three times in a row, consciously and deliberately, it will be one of the elements that give your life structure, in your autonomous mental planner. You won't be able to cut it out, except if you decide to do this just as consciously and deliberately as you decided to adopt it. When Wednesday evening comes round, an automatic internal reminder will tell you that the next day is a day in your Stabilization programme, the programme that's part of your life plan.

Whenever I meet someone who tells me that they've lost weight with my method but can feel the weight going back on, I ask them if they're following their Protein Thursdays, and the reply is always NO. The day that you too give up the protection Protein Thursday offers, you'll be entering a high-risk zone.

From that moment on, there are three possible scenarios:

1. You'll have learnt how to feed yourself – and having changed the way you're 'programmed' to eat, you'll have turned into a different person.
2. Or you'll have adopted a far more active lifestyle which will offset your vulnerability to weight, and you'll

stabilize as long as you keep active. But if you start leading a sedentary lifestyle, you'll put weight back on.
3. Or the pounds will go back on, more or less slowly – but surely.

The reality is quite simple: if after losing weight you don't want to regain it, something has to change in the way you eat. Protein Thursdays will spearhead this change.

There's nothing magical about opting for Thursday. Apart from being a day in the middle of the week, it was an arbitrary choice. On the other hand, what isn't arbitrary is that it's fixed. When I started introducing this high-security day, I simply asked my patients to follow 'one day a week', without specifying any particular day. They all started off enthusiastically but few kept going. They'd keep putting it off to the next day and eventually gave it up altogether. This brought home to me that, to make sure the measure was followed, it was better to set a fixed day, so that it becomes a non-negotiable necessity, prescribed by an outside authority. So I chose Thursday and immediately this radically changed how it was adopted and its effects.

When I examine daily weight chart statistics for my patients in Stabilization, I can see the importance of Thursday for getting everything back on track. Indeed from Friday to Wednesday evening, the graphs go up by half an ounce or so, a modest addition due to the little extras spread out over the week. If it has been a very enjoyable week, weight gain can reach or even exceed an ounce by the time you weigh yourself before eating on Thursday. But by the time you weigh yourself again on Friday morning, this small surplus will have automatically disappeared.

You can see just how important it is not to let any apparently harmless drifting go on for any longer than a week.

But do be careful! A protein day gives you extremely good results, but only provided you follow it to the letter.

If, for some reason beyond your control, you're unable to keep to your Protein Thursday you can shift it to Wednesday or Friday. The interval for effectiveness between two days of proteins is one week, but there's no real problem if occasionally you have to change it to six or eight days instead.

For how long should you do Protein Thursdays?
If you've lost around a stone (7 kilos), my advice is to do it for as long as possible, and for at least seven months after Consolidation. Apart from its role in stabilizing your weight, one day of proteins a week is in itself a great way of protecting your body and mind, a sort of cure to cleanse your body and let it rest. By doing this, your liver, digestive tract and pancreas enjoy a highly beneficial short break to recuperate. As for your kidneys, contrary to the stories invented by the world of sugar, they're made to process proteins and eliminate the waste products, just like the kidneys of any carnivores on the planet. What

kidneys most fear is sugar, since they're not made to deal with it – which explains why 80 per cent of people on dialysis are diabetic.

If you've lost over a stone, I'm asking you to incorporate it permanently into your life. Over 2¼ stone, Thursdays play a crucial role: ignoring them means regaining the weight you lost. Don't wait to learn from bitter experience. Tell yourself that it's part of your life, just as for some people Friday is a day for fish, or they never eat pork or gluten, and others are vegetarians or even vegans.

A 20-minute Walk Every Day and No Lifts or Escalators

A 20-minute walk

Sceptical, you ask me how 20 minutes of physical activity that uses up so few calories can help keep weight off.

As far as physical effort goes, walking doesn't burn up many calories. This is true, but walking has other benefits. This 20-minute walk is aimed at the physically inactive, for whom exercise is deemed a waste of time and boring into the bargain. To them I'd like to prove the contrary.

Why walking?

Firstly, because walking is mankind's biological signature. Man ceased being a great ape when he stood up and stopped using all four limbs to move. This posture led to walking on the hind limbs and thereafter to all the other mutations that the human species has undergone until now. Standing up on both legs, with face and eyes

342

peering out over the high grasses of the savanna, our distant ancestors could spot both prey and predators from afar. Which left this creature's arms free, as it came closer to becoming human. The head no longer needed to be supported by powerful cervical muscles. This was the start of the development of the back of the skull and the brain. A dialogue was established between the brain and hands, neural connections multiplied. A huge number of mutations resulted in the birth of language, consciousness and man's supreme resources.

Walking is right at the heart of the human phenomenon. It would be most unwise to see it merely as a way of getting around or burning up calories. This fundamental activity is embedded in our brain's 'primitive software', hard-wired as being necessary and therefore 'rewarded' by the brain which owes it so much, as far as evolution is concerned.

Another thing is that walking or a slow/semi-fast jog is the only exercise that doesn't make you feel hungry. What's the point of spending an hour at the gym, sweating over machines, if hunger, which knows no mercy, drives you to eat the equivalent of what you've just burnt off? I love swimming, I go diving and snorkelling. I know full well that after an hour or two in the water I could devour a whole meal. Knowing this and to avoid carbs, I often take along a couple of yoghurts, an oat bran galette and a flask of gazpacho.

The energy used up by walking varies depending on its speed and intensity. If brisk, walking can burn up to 300 calories an hour, or 100 calories per 20 minutes. This doesn't appear very much, but over a year, it becomes a useful amount.

As an automatic behaviour, walking also improves creativity. Whenever I have to do some important thinking, I go for a walk. The feeling of being disconnected from the rest of my body as it moves forward all on its own enables me to concentrate better. Many artists and even scientists know this; they go for a walk because it frees up thought and intuition.

Walking also has the advantage that you can do it anywhere and at any time – in town or in the country, on a beach, up a mountain or as a proper hike. You can combine walking with a cultural or tourist outing, you can walk at any time of the day or night, before and especially *after* mealtimes.

Walking costs nothing. So if it's done in a gym on a treadmill it loses some of its meaning and symbolic force.

Another advantage is that walking doesn't make you sweat. So you can walk in whatever outfit you choose!

Walking is the only exercise an obese person can take that is risk-free. What's more, it spares them withdrawal and social discrimination, which is very important.

Finally, and this is crucial, provided it's done for at least 20 minutes a day, walking produces a very beneficial effect on the brain. For a long time this phenomenon intrigued the international scientific community. Neuroscience has now been able to prove that **regular walking generates an equally regular secretion of**

serotonin and of such intensity that the serotonin produced naturally can match mainstream anti-depressant treatments. Isn't that amazing?

And you need the pleasure that walking can bring you. Before, you used to go looking for this pleasure in food, which didn't suit your body as you became overweight. Now you know what your brain is looking for, give it some pleasure . . . but without the pounds!

So go walking every day for at least 20 minutes. If you're still doubtful about serotonin's role and how good walking is for you, I recommend you read *Spark!: The Revolutionary New Science of Exercise and the Brain* by John J. Ratey and Eric Hagerman (Quercus, 2010).

Giving up lifts and escalators

Here, as with Protein Thursdays and your daily 20-minute walk, it's about setting up a simple, easy and really effective ritual to protect you.

As far as energy goes, in the course of a day, at home, visiting people, at work, at train stations and in the underground, you'll climb a dozen or so floors, i.e. at least 70 calories. This may not seem much to you, but add them to the 100 calories from your daily walk and you'll have burnt up enough energy to absorb a couple of food whims – whims that will almost certainly be carb foods, which you'll therefore need to neutralize urgently. You'll need to burn their sugar up before your pancreas gets round to secreting insulin, the number one cause for storing fat.

However, there's another reason why it's good to walk up the stairs. In our world of comfort and immobility, this ritual imposes on us some rather unenticing physical activity. So why would I encourage you to adopt it? First of all, after two weeks of taking the stairs, your quadricep muscles – the ones that lift your body up on to each step – get stronger and bigger, thus making it easier and then pleasant for you to climb up. This means that in your own way you're tackling one of the root causes for being overweight – lack of exercise. You've stopped giving into the siren calls for total comfort and ease that our consumerist society constantly bombards you with. Instead, you're embracing a natural physical activity, which costs nothing.

Seen this way, refusing to use lifts and escalators is a sensible thing to do. You're not only using your body, but you're also reminding our consumption-based society that you exist and you're not totally in thrall to its interests. You're voting against – with your legs and with your new-found fitness! The advantages of technological innovation are increasingly meagre when we look at the damage and harm they can cause. Many thinkers who reflect on happiness, and I'd like to be considered one of them, believe that we've gone past our limits, that the drawbacks far exceed any gains, that modern life doesn't make us as happy as it claims. Yes, let's embrace science and technological innovation but by applying critical reason. However, this fascinating debate on happiness and what creates it is too much of a digression, so let's get back to what interests you.

Stabilization and controlling your weight imply that you refuse to use lifts and escalators. You're on the ground floor of a block of flats, someone is waiting for you on the fourth, and you're halfway between the first few steps of the stairway on one side and the lift door on the other. This is the moment of choice. If you opt for the stairs, your determination takes you forward, you can feel some pride – I'd even goes as far as saying a victory – and the situation remains under your control. However, if you choose the lift, you're undermining your determination, you're eroding the ritual. You'll say I'm making a mountain out of a molehill, that it's nothing, just a detail. Well, it isn't. When you stop weighing yourself, you'll tell yourself that it's just a detail too, whereas in reality, you're starting to compromise. And tomorrow, it'll be the turn of your Protein Thursdays; you'll shift them, forget them and then you'll give them up altogether. People who've put weight back on started compromising over what they thought was just a detail.

Keep in mind that, in their natural environment, all living creatures are protected by an automatic, biological system of regulation. However, once they leave this environment, as we humans have done, the system is lost and we have to make a point of taking control over it.

By choosing the stairs, you're taking up a position. You've grasped the crux of your problem about being overweight; you're putting up a symbolic barrier against regaining weight. But you're also taking up a position with regard to society. You're making plain your desire

347

to remain human, within a society that couldn't give a hoot about your health. This simple gesture of walking up the stairs then takes on another dimension; it becomes part of a far wider, collective cause and combat. Give it a go.

3 Tablespoons of Oat Bran a Day

I've already explained what's important about oat bran; I related how I came across it and made it part of my original method, then my second front. Just like konjac in all its guises, oat bran is a 'Robin Hood' food that steals from over-rich foods.

In this final Stabilization phase, apart from working to fill our stomachs, make us feel full and sneak away calories from the intestines, oat bran joins forces with Protein Thursdays, walking and using the stairs. It's another point of reference and a ritual to protect your weight. And if Protein Thursdays, walking and taking the stairs are part of the restrictiveness you've conquered, oat bran is a source of pleasure and culinary inspiration. Carry on making your galettes, your muffins, pizza bases and bread, but do your utmost to stay with this protective food.

I'd like to finish by honestly saying that I've never met anyone who had failed to stabilize their weight following this Stabilization programme with its three measures. On the other hand, I've met a great many who chose not to follow it and consequently they put back some or all of the weight they'd lost.

If, after the work we've done together, you join the category of stabilized dieters who are forever cured of being overweight, I'd ask that you please let me know.

And if, despite everything, you still put weight back on, there is a solution.

The Flexible Response System

The Flexible Response system is a technique to protect your stabilization. I devised it to rescue anyone who had let their weight slip, despite the protective guidance that Stabilization offers. Once a woman has lost weight, she usually feels better inside her skin and her head, she prefers her new figure, finds herself more attractive and lighter, and she's proud of having managed to get rid of her unwanted pounds. So she's firmly resolved to maintain her new weight. As for men, I'm always surprised at how happy and proud they are, too, at having slimmed down and got rid of the paunch that was depressing them.

And yet . . .

Looking at all the results from traditional diets, the international statistics are devastating: 95 per cent of people who lose weight put it back on again. WHY?

To my mind, there are two main reasons for this general failure:

1. The first is to do with calorie-counting, which runs completely counter to the psychology of overweight

people. When dealing with food, their senses and emotions are involved, and this is diametrically opposed to arithmetic and calorie calculations. When you love, you don't count whatever it is that you love! And the time spent on all this counting eats into motivation, and all the quicker the less convincing the results are.

2. The second is to do with the astonishing fact that there's no proper structured stabilization programme. There may be loads of weight-loss diets, but I haven't yet found a reliable, well-thought-out and carefully contructed method for the post-diet period. Which is one of the reasons why I've been so insistent that you follow the instructions I've given you. This Stabiliza-tion programme is made to keep you going over the long term, and avoid the number one pitfall with weight-loss dieting.

It was to fill this gap that I worked out the Flexible Response, an ultimate fallback system to 'protect the protection'.

I sincerely hope that you won't need it, but just remem-ber that even if you do stumble, everything has been put in place to catch you.

If there's any weight regain, the Flexible Response system is there to protect you with its look-out post and a rapid reaction force. In practice, you've got four succes-sive lines of defence that pop up one after the other should the one before give way. They are there to rescue you and get you back to your True Weight.

A Basic Condition: Weigh Yourself Every Day!

The whole Flexible Response system is based around weighing yourself daily. Rid yourself of the absurd, obscurantist prejudice that makes people believe that weighing yourself daily is obsessive behaviour. Not only is this untrue, but it defies common sense, logic and most of all achieving results.

Everyone who is part of my group of permanently stabilized patients weighs themselves each morning. How could you stabilize your weight without monitoring what's happening to it? As a rule, people who stop weighing themselves are afraid to step on the scales, because they fear seeing confirmation of what they already sense or know.

So weigh yourself every morning, in the same outfit.

Ideally you should record your weight on a piece of paper or, better still, on an Excel spreadsheet, which you can then use to create a chart. This means you can visualize what is happening with your weight and, believe me, this is really important. As long as you're monitoring your weight, you'll remain on track; you'll know where you really are with your stabilization. At the first sign of any weight regain, get going with the Flexible Responses. If you breach the first barrier, a second one will go up straightaway, and this will continue.

Take Action Quickly – It's Much Easier Not to Put on a Pound Than It Is to Lose It!

Time is against you, as far as both your metabolism and behaviour patterns are concerned. The longer you take to react, the more entrenched your weight gain becomes and the more it will withstand any dieting or exercise you use to get rid of it. So once your celebration meal is over, go for a brisk one-hour walk straightaway. This way you'll stand a good chance of preventing the calories you've just ingested from turning into fat.

If you wait until the next day to do something, it'll be a little less easy but still possible.

A week later, the surplus calories will already have been stored away in your reserves, but only in your surface fat, and once again you can still react and get results.

A month later, this fat will be lost deep down in your reserves and infinitely more difficult to access. Only a strong, structured diet will be able to get the situation under control.

An image to help you understand: compare your over-eating to painting a wall. If you want to wipe the paint off as soon as you've applied it, it's easy because it's fresh and still wet. The longer you wait, the more the paint sets, and once it has dried completely a cloth won't do the job. You'll need a scraper and plenty of elbow grease to get rid of it.

So weigh yourself and do something quickly. But that's not all.

In practice, if you've put some weight back on, it's because you've dropped your guard, forgotten or neglected your protective trident: **Protein Thursdays** + **stairs and 20-minute walk** + **oat bran**. It's because you've shirked from one, two or three of these measures that are there to tether you to your True Weight.

So just how do you react? There are two possible ways, one that's simple, technical, immediate and tactical. The other goes deeper and requires a little more thought; it's strategic and connected with how you redeploy your sources of self-fulfilment.

Let's start with the immediate response.

Your Position – Armed and Ready

First and foremost, you need a reference point, the north position on your stabilization compass. This reference point is the weight you've just lost, the difference between your initial weight and the weight you attained, the weight you want to get back to and stabilize at.

As you don't have the body or lifestyle of a robot, keep a margin for manoeuvre of about 3¼ pounds (1.5 kilos). With its variations in water and food, this is your body's breathing space. Also, you're bound to get invited out to friends, birthday celebrations, parties and business lunches, so your body needs to breathe socially as well.

As long as you don't go beyond this margin, everything is okay, you're still on track. But once you pass this boundary, you're starting to drift and you need your scales to point it out to you. Don't trust your clothes or your belts;

it's all too easy to blame a pair of jeans that have shrunk in the wash, or to pull your tummy in to fasten a belt. WEIGH YOURSELF!

First Response

Beyond 3¼ pounds, you need to take action.

GO BACK TO YOUR PROTEIN THURSDAYS because you've certainly given them up. Better still, make it a double – add a second day of proteins, the Wednesday or the Friday, either but you need two consecutive days, and carry on until you're back down to your correct weight.

Start taking the stairs again. You can't have been using them, otherwise you wouldn't have regained those pounds. And also WALK AN EXTRA 15 MINUTES.

And if, as is also quite likely, you've given up your oat bran, go back to it and increase it to 5 tablespoons per day.

Finally, drink more: increase your intake to 2 litres (3½ pints) of still water, with a very low mineral content.

Second Response

What if you've regained a third of the pounds you lost? For example, after losing 1½ stone you've put ½ stone back on. Attack with two consecutive days of proteins, go back to the beginning of the Nutritional Staircase until you lose the rest, and then go through a week of Consolidation again.

Here too you need to start using the stairs again and WALK AN EXTRA 30 MINUTES each day.

Go back to 1½ tablespoons of oat bran until you're stabilized again.

PP	PP	x Nutritional Staircase weeks until you reach your True Weight	1 week Consolidation	Go back to Stabilization

Third Response

If you've put back more than half of what you lost, you're losing the benefit of all your hard work. Since the regain is recent, you can still hope to shift it again fairly easily. But you've already stretched things as far as they'll go. This moment is CRUCIAL, don't let it pass by. If you wait a moment longer, this all-too-risky day will tip you over into the 'irreparable' zone. 'Irreparable' quite simply means permanent regain.

Begin by alternating one day of proteins with one day of proteins + vegetables and a third day of proteins + vegetables + one piece of fruit. Follow this three-day alternating pattern three times in a row, i.e. for nine days. Then go back to the Nutritional Staircase week until you've dropped down to your True Weight again. Spend five days in Consolidation per 2 pounds you've just lost again.

As with the second response, go back to using the stairs and in addition WALK 30 EXTRA MINUTES every day.

Stick with 1½ tablespoons of oat bran until you've stabilized.

And, most importantly, remember that despite your good results and your great success, you nevertheless put half of this weight back on. So never make the mistake of being complacent; regain is always possible. You opened a door when you put on weight and it will never, ever quite close again all on its own. So be on your guard and take action quickly.

3 cycles of PP–PV–PV+1 Fruit	x Nutritional Staircase	5 days Consolidation/ 2lb lost	Return to Stabilization

Fourth Response

If you regain three-quarters of what you lost, you're no longer looking at some accidental occurence but at repeat offending. Should this happen to you, it's because there's a flaw or failing in the way you make yourself feel fulfilled which is compelling you to seek comfort and reward from food.

Either you're going through a vulnerable period when you're too susceptible to life's difficulties, or you're buckling under the strain, unable to cope with the stress, which is quite different.

If your real difficulties are temporary, however great they may be (for example, a divorce, being laid off work or immediate money problems), then you just need to wait until things calm down and you can cope with life again. Until this happens, go back to the Consolidation phase, but with two protein days instead of one.

And as soon as your fortunes start to look up, return to the second front and go right back to the beginning with weeks on the Nutritional Staircase. Once you've attained your True Weight, move into the Consolidation phase. Next, commit once again to your permanent stabilization, and this time take on board a valuable lesson from your repeat offending so that, should you ever encounter turbulent times again, you can look after yourself.

If your weight regain isn't really connected to any identifiable obstacle and has more to do with your hypersensitivity and a vulnerability that's unique to you, this means that you need to think about how to change the way you get comfort and reward. You need to find ways of producing pleasure to compensate that don't make you fat. For years, I've been working to devise a tool to achieve life's main goal – finding pleasure in being alive – which we call happiness. Up until now this fundamental question has been left to philosophers, moralists and religious thinkers. But the answers they provide are always more theoretical than practical. Just email me if you'd like me to let you know when this method becomes available (you'll find my address on page 400).

Even if you don't wish to make any further changes in how you find compensation, I advise you not to throw in the towel altogether. Because as long as you're still battling against your weight problems and the risks, it means you're taking action and not giving way to the stress of the situation. So I ask that you do just one thing – go for a 30-minute walk every day and then for a whole hour on Saturday and Sunday, striding as energetically as you can. Within a few days, I KNOW that you'll have secreted enough serotonin to feel able to make ONE DAY A WEEK of proteins your sanctuary. And as soon as you feel up to it, repeat the second front right from the beginning.

So there you are, you've now got everything I can give you to help you control your weight problem. You have the means to decide which attack profile is most able to lead you to victory. I created this second front for people with a different profile, having in all humility realized that my first front couldn't help all overweight people.

Now it's up to you to do something.

III

FIGHTING AT YOUR SIDE

Flashback

Looking back over the course my life has taken, I have the feeling of having been born with what was going to become my *raison d'être* – my fight to overcome the weight scourge. I was born at a turning point in mankind's history. Was it coincidence, destiny? There has been spectacular progress in the development of technologies to connect us as well as in neuroscientific research, alongside intense acceleration in the economy. And it is from this world which is getting ever richer, but also ever more artificial and stressful, that weight problems, obesity and diabetes have emerged.

In 1944, weight problems didn't exist. In France, there weren't enough overweight or obese people to form a *composite* group. Of course some people were overweight and even obese, but they were few and far between.

In 1960, my first year as a medical student, there was uproar when the number of obese people in France reached 1 million for the first time! Today there are 7 million.

It seems to me that this record was always deliberately overlooked: nothing before 1944, 1 million obese people in 1960, 7 million today among 27 million who are overweight. Nevertheless, these figures pose the question of weight problems being a lifestyle problem, created by the choices society makes. You'd have to be peculiarly insincere not to concede that weight problems are a disease of civilization.

In 1966, I finished studying medicine, wrote my thesis and then started specializing in neurology. In the mornings I worked in a hospital in Garches, in the west of Paris, and in the afternoons I saw patients in a small surgery. I discovered both the tragic suffering in neurology, and the art of being a general practitioner.

In my local surgery, I was to come across a man who unwittingly would change the course of my life. He published poetry and I liked him. He was obese and one day he asked me to help him lose weight. I've told this story often and I'll carry on telling it because it's why I'm here with you. He asked me to help him shed the six stone that were ruining his life. As I wasn't a nutritionist at the time, I declined.

He kept insisting and finally came out with this surprising sentence: 'Give me any diet you want, ban any foods you want, but not meat.' Our chap loved meat. And his plea contained the only possible reply. So I prescribed him lean meat and plenty of water for five days. And the results were unbelievable: he lost 11 pounds.

It was because of this single and spectacular case that I made up my mind to specialize in nutrition instead of neurology.

I then worked in a department run by Professor Gilbert Dreyfus, the main centre for nutrition, under the wing of Dr Marcel Zara, who would later sign my first book. For three years, I was taught the same principles about nutrition as all the others who became the main players in the field then and now. The theory practised at the time was based around calories; counting and calculating what was consumed and what was used to keep the body functioning.

According to the prevailing theory, an obese person could become less obese simply by reducing the number of calories consumed. And there were three diets for this: the 1,500-calorie, the 1,200-calorie and the 900-calorie diets.

In 1970, when I proudly put up my nutritionist's plaque outside my surgery, it was not without nostalgia for general medicine. I was now going to devote myself to nutrition, weight problems, obesity and diabetes, and to thyroid conditions, Dr Zara's area of specialism.

And I used these three low-calorie diets with great enthusiasm. However, despite my commitment and huge desire to achieve results, they were disappointing. Laborious, slow and, then once achieved, very tenuous. As soon as the support, guidance and close relationship between me and my patients ended, their weight gain was systematic.

After so much hope, effort and commitment and after investing so much time on both sides, we found that we had reached a dead end. Like many of my nutritionist friends and colleagues, I could have contented myself with persisting in following the conventional approach. But being by nature someone who rises to a challenge, I wasn't afraid of stepping outside of a reassuring framework founded on authority, or of battling passionately against the odds, when required.

I'd just stopped working with neurology patients whose enormous suffering had at times overwhelmed me. And I was now discovering a deep affinity with my overweight patients. They were touching as they searched for help and kindness that I felt all too ready to give them. And, unable to do any better for them, I was beside myself. Doctors like to cure, that's their best reward!

At that time, medicine had no interest in weight problems, let alone preventing them. It was only concerned with obesity and severe, late-onset complications without any connection being made to the patient's weight problem background. Being overweight was even seen as a 'female' problem, i.e. inconsequential and insignificant. Magazines would run front-page features on women's 'seasonal eagerness' to rid themselves of their unwanted pounds for the summer. It was the done thing to make much of the jovial, likeable '*bon viveur*'. The suffering of living in an unloved body, feeling unattractive and marginalized was ignored. As for what was causing weight problems, nobody even really asked the question.

I found that the vast majority of my patients experienced a real sense of discomfort, and that they had felt it before growing fat. They ate to silence their misery. Foods with sugar, fat and salt brought them comfort. I didn't know what to do until I recalled the wonderful experiment with my publisher who'd so loved his rare steaks. I knew that if he had managed to lose weight really quickly, while still eating plentifully, it was because he ate all those very high-quality proteins.

Based on this, I established what would become the Attack phase in my future method. For short periods of targeted dieting, I prescribed these high-protein foods. This meant leaving calorie-counting behind, since using it didn't achieve the results I was looking for.

Suddenly everything changed and the results were staggering. My patients were surprised and delighted. Their motivation didn't waver and I shared in their enthusiasm and joy. We were on the way to meeting the challenge, to winning the wager. It was truly exciting. I was forging a way ahead as a pathfinder, an explorer, a searcher.

My patients didn't have access to such a wide range of high-protein foods as we have available today. It was more or less the range the hunter-gatherers had in the Paleolithic era! No low-fat dairy products, no seafood sticks, no tuna in brine, no low-fat sliced ham, turkey or chicken, no bresaola, no vegetable proteins such as tofu, seitan or tempeh. I hadn't yet come across oat bran or konjac and its calorie-free pasta and rice. However, my patients had only one thing in mind – losing weight. The rest or what would follow afterwards didn't seem to bother or interest them. Once they'd slimmed down, we took leave of one another, satisfied and feeling that our mission was accomplished. Unfortunately, this weight loss wasn't maintained; it turned out to be as unstable as what the calorie-restricted diets achieved. In the six months afterwards, they'd become fat again. I couldn't just stand by helplessly and accept the situation; I had to keep moving on to find something better.

This drove me to offer a follow-up to the lightning-quick results obtained with the **Attack phase**. My patients had been so satisfied with what they'd lost so quickly that they were more than happy to try the experiment I suggested to them. **This was how I introduced the Cruise phase**. Its role was to calm metabolic action down, while also prolonging weight loss, but at a steadier rhythm.

So I kept all the Attack phase high-protein foods, still with the magic words 'as much as you want', and to them I added all vegetables, except any starchy ones. Here was a very wide range of natural, healthy foods, packed with vitamins, mineral salts and fibre, yet sufficiently low-carb not to jeopardize the results achieved in the Attack phase. This allowed me to deploy my method over longer periods and therefore treat heavily overweight and obese patients.

At the same time, I became passionately interested in prehistoric times. Through primitive man we can see the fundamental matrix of human beings before it became entangled within our infinitely complex modern culture. Primitive man is a mirror of ourselves, and I could see this behavioural matrix at work everywhere, and in particular in my patients. The inspiring courses taught by

Professor Leroi-Gourhan at the Collège de France and those given by Professor de Lumley at the Musée de l'Homme on prehistoric man's diet, and on the diet of indigenous peoples still alive in the first half of the twentieth century, bore out my strategy. Adding vegetables to proteins created a dietary framework very close to that of the hunter-gatherers.

Take a look at the table below, which tells us a lot about food in prehistoric times. It was compiled by Professor Gilles Delluc, a friend and former pupil of Professor Leroi-Gourhan:

AUSTRALO-PITHECUS	FIRST MEN	MIDDLE, LATER PALEOLITHIC	PREHISTORY AND HISTORY	TODAY
tubers, roots . . .	tubers, roots . . .	tubers, roots . . .	tubers, roots . . .	vegetables, fruit little plant fibre
		depending on the climate	cereals and dairy products	fast sugars
				cereals and bread
		meat products (hunting and fishing)		dairy products (saturated fatty acids)
insects	meat (carrion and hunting)		meat products (cattle rearing, hunting, fishing)	meat (saturated fatty acids) and fish
small animals				

Extract from *La Nutrition préhistorique* (Prehistoric nutrition) by Gilles Delluc.

From the Paleolithic era until the 1940s, i.e. for 99.5 per cent of the time humans have existed, we've eaten game, fish and wild fibrous plants, food that was hard to come by. Then over about 60 years or so, i.e. 0.5 per cent of our evolution, we've turned into a population made up mostly of city dwellers and people who lead sedentary lives. Nowadays, we're affected or threatened on a large scale by obesity, weight problems, diabetes in the elderly, high blood pressure, abnormal blood lipids, coronary disease, strokes and probably certain cancers – the diseases afflicting us in our twenty-first century.

The conclusion was glaringly obvious and confirmed the choices I'd made: the dietary model genetically programmed inside us, and which had remained unchanged since we first came into being, was that of the hunter-gatherer. We had to go back to it, take inspiration from it – that was the key. The Cruise phase, when it introduced the gatherer's vegetables alongside the hunter's proteins from the Attack phase, gave the human body all the essential food it needed with its healthy frugality.

And, the results for the Cruise phase were convincing, which came as no surprise to me.

Had I achieved my goal? Not yet. Because, once again, my patients' weight remained unstable. Often they didn't regain the whole amount and it came back over a longer period, a year instead of a few months, but it still came back. This really saddened me as a doctor because I had the impression of building on sand and of only temporarily improving an incurable chronic illness. I had to succeed in getting weight to stabilize.

So I then aked myself two questions for which there was no answer in my medical discipline.

I wondered if it was better to have managed to lose and maintain the new weight for a year than to just continue being overweight. And whether the fact that a person spent a year a stone and a half lighter would help reduce the risks connected with obesity over the long term, and whether it was beneficial, neutral or in fact disadvantageous? At the time I thought that there was no point in losing weight only to regain it and that this could even give the body an extra opportunity to develop its resistance to dieting.

Today, I've shifted my position on this point. If it is true that successive diets are often slower and less successful than the first ones, this has more to do with psychological than metabolic impediments. Even if your morale is the same, you don't follow a diet as well the second time round, because it boils down to motivation. This said, I've met a great many patients, and monitored readers and website users, who've come back to my first front having failed to follow it properly the first time, and often they've got far better results than with their first attempt. Experience has taught me that living for one, two or three years a stone or two lighter reduces and delays the onset of the risks that come with being overweight. Like a smoker who gets through a packet a day, giving up for a year or two means the bronchial tubes and arteries don't get clogged up during that time. And this always has to be better for their health.

The other question was the speed of weight loss. Intuitively, we're inclined to think that a very fast, effective diet leads to more instability and weight regain than a slow diet. In fact, it's the exact opposite. Studies carried out in the United States have provided clear proof. To achieve significant weight loss, a slow and laborious diet erodes motivation to such an extent that it has become exhausted at the very point when decisive effort is required to stabilize the new weight.

The crucial problem about how to stabilize my patients still remained. It took me many long years to develop the two Consolidation and weight Stabilization phases.

The post-diet period is your whole life, i.e. the rest of your life without any extra pounds or any health risks from being overweight. It was vital for my patients, and for me absolutely necessary that I succeeded here. For me, the research was exciting and stimulating because I really don't believe that anyone is doomed to remain overweight.

However, to keep weight off for good, several obstacles have to be overcome. It was also to help you that I devised this second front. Increased appetite, reduction in energy used and maximum extraction of the calories from food ingested – these all combine to undermine any weight loss that has been achieved. Lessons had to be drawn from all of this. Firewalls had to be set up to fight these natural reactions.

So I worked out how long this vulnerability lasts and realized that the risk of rebound is connected with the size of the weight loss: approximately five days for every pound lost. Based on this, I was able to give precise, simple and concrete instructions to guide and encourage you to keep going until the threat of rebound dies away.

By devising a more sophisticated weight calculation than the BMI, I was able to estimate any individual's True Weight and make it a sensible and sustainable target.

Once consolidation was achieved, there had to be stabilization. And I had to ensure that eating was as free and normal as possible. I realized that with freedom and rediscovered independence, there'd be a few lapses, and so **three simple instructions** were put in place that have to be followed lifelong to protect you from regaining weight. These were **Protein Thursdays**, **oat bran**, and the **20-minute walk**. Lastly, I explained to you how these three measures are here for you, just like this second front, which marks a milestone as I fight with you, at your side.

Right Of Reply

Despite the weight pandemic, nutritional diets currently have a bad press. In November 2010, ANSES (the French Agency for Food, Environmental and Occupational Health and Safety) was asked to report on the risks involved with the 15 most commonly used diets in France. In general, it emphasized that 'following a diet, regardless which diet, is no trivial matter and has unwanted side effects'. It pointed out variations in micronutrient and fibre intake, as well as a range of metabolic changes related to the proportion of nutrients provided by each diet. This is stating the blindingly obvious! By definition, any weight-loss diet that reduces food intake will reduce micronutrient and fibre intake proportionately, reducing stool volume and speed of digestion accordingly.

But when it really comes to it, what do these side effects matter when we're faced with a toxic onslaught of obesity and diabetes, so often associated with the risk of heart attack, going blind, successive amputations, kidney failure and spending the end of your days on dialysis, which is about as bad as it gets? Who is being taken for a ride here? On the one hand, some mild disorders, and on the other 2.8 million deaths each year worldwide directly caused by obesity, weight problems and diabetes, which WHO defines as a scourge and the planet's main preventable health risk.

ANSES is an administrative agency, which was asked to carry out a task by its supervisory authorities, who more than likely come under perfectly legitimate pressure from economic forces – whose interests are not primarily focused on protecting our health.

However, as ANSES has not been the only body to challenge my method, I'd like to discuss some of this criticism. And I'd like to start by saying that it rarely comes from anyone who has followed my diet right to the end. Criticism comes mostly from lobbies – for them a successful dieter equates to losing a consumer, i.e. a customer. Over the past three years the sugar, white flour and snack-food industries have seen their sales decline. They recruit their spokespersons among the very nutritionists who have suffered most from my method's popularity. Yes, I did overturn the calorie dogma, get results, point out the damage from sugar and achieve great success. Good enough reasons to provoke jealousy and hostility. However, you're my readers and entitled to hear my arguments. And like any citizen, I'm exercising my right to reply to such attacks, which may sow seeds of doubt in your minds.

I maintain that creating a diet is about taking care of you.

• *I've been criticized for using too many high-protein foods.*

I advocate proteins because I believe that they offer considerable benefits in helping us fight weight problems, since they have *absolutely no*, and yes I did say *absolutely no*, downside. In the first year of medicine, students learn that too many carbs results in diabetes and weight problems and too many saturated fats in cardio-vascular risk. However, proteins do not result in any pathology.

If we list their advantages, proteins are the most filling foods, whereas sugar is addictive and fats neutral. Proteins are highly thermogenic – a third of their calories get burnt up during digestion, while very few of the calories in carbs and fats do. Proteins chase water away and help prevent water retention; carbs and fats do not.

For anyone wanting to lose weight, these three benefits play a significant role.

Moreover, if I favour proteins, I bestow even more importance on vegetables. For years, I've been constantly repeating my recommendation to eat them 'as much as you can'.

Proteins and vegetables combined comprise the natural basis of our human diet.

• *It's been said that proteins might be dangerous for the kidneys.*

Not only is this incorrect, but the exact opposite is true! Let's look at the facts. A great number of epidemiological studies show that there's no risk for healthy people. Furthermore, Dr M.M. Poplawski (Mount Sinai School of Medicine, New York) has proven, clinically, functionally and biologically that kidney conditions (including the most serious ones) resulting from diabetes could be reversed by following a ketogenic (carb-free) diet made up solely of proteins and fats. The vast majority of cases of kidney disease that require dialysis are diabetic, due to glucose toxicity for the kidneys, as well as for the eyes, heart, brain arteries and lower limbs. I've personally treated 60 patients who followed my diet with only one normal kidney. I monitored them very closely, carried out regular blood tests and never saw any disturbance in their kidney function. The only nutrient that can damage the kidneys through overconsumption is carbs, with over-consumption of sugar leading to diabetes.

• *It's been said that my diet produces weight loss too quickly.*

Why move slowly when you can go faster? What's better about being slow? Psychologically, being able to diet quickly spurs people on and drives motivation, and is the mainspring for beginning, following, succeeding with and consolidating a weight-loss programme. But prejudice is deep-rooted. Are we really meant to dilly-dally, deprive ourselves for no good reason and be miserable for ages? This is pointless, demotivating and unjustifiable.

• *It's been said that there's weight regain with my diet.*

This is sometimes the case with people who don't follow my Post-Diet. Inevitably, the same causes have the same effects; these people put weight back on because they revert to eating too many carbs and fats. However, there's no weight regain whenever my method (first or second front) is followed to the letter during the Consolidation and Stabilization phases, and my three precautionary measures (walking + oat bran + Protein Thursdays) are adopted for life. My diet is the only one that takes care of the post-diet period, with a nutritionally balanced plat-form as reference point and the minimal restriction of three corrective measures. What's more, this second front attaches even greater importance to Consolidation and Stabilization. One of the reasons for devising it was that I wanted to further bolster the post-diet period.

• *My diet is criticized for not being balanced.*

This is a specious argument. Anyone who has grown fat has done so by eating in an **unbalanced** way, with too many carbs and fats. To lose weight, they have to correct this imbalance and go into reverse while losing weight – as few carbs and fats as possible, that's what my method is based on. Offering them a balanced diet right away would only maintain them at their current weight; they'd be unable to shift the unwanted pounds. And, yes, by all means go back to a balanced diet afterwards. In my diet, which is similar to the Cretan diet, no nutrient is missing. Having said this, the second front offers a solution to all of you who wish to continue eating almost all foods.

• My diet is criticized for . . . being a diet!

After decades of diet crazes, a 'down with diets' trend has recently emerged. It would have you believe that it's possible to slim without dieting, which is utter nonsense. Simply eating a balanced diet won't make you lose weight. It's not the first time that we've heard similar talk. Unfortunately, come the aftermath there's always a rude awakening.

Despite these challenges, I remain confident because there's a solution, and a comprehensive one at that. And it's you who has it. You alone are capable of making things happen. You've already done it when so many of you used my method, spreading the word all over the world. You understood my message and advice. Faced with resignation all around us, here is a bright glimmer of hope. With you and for you, I'd like to go further still and not be happy simply to see the prevalence of weight problems slow down, even if there is a definite slowing down. We've got to put an actual stop to this trend, and do all we can to reverse it.

And this will happen at an individual level, person by person. This is why I've opened this second front, to extend the scope of our fight and persuade more over-weight people to take action.

Far too often minor amounts of excess weight, below $1\frac{1}{2}$ stone, are overlooked. And yet, 100 per cent of obese people have at some point in their lives had under $1\frac{1}{2}$ stone to lose. And if they'd been helped at that point in time, their medical and personal complications could have been avoided. It was the same with diabetes; for decades, people talked about 'minor diabetes', which didn't get treated. Nowadays, the watchword for diabetes treatment is: 'take action as early, as quickly and as effectively as possible'. I'd really like the same to happen with 'minor' amounts of excess weight, i.e. for action to be taken as early, as quickly and as effectively as possible!

• *I've been criticized for concerning myself with people's happiness, whether they wanted me to or not, and for presenting fat and obese people as being unhappy.*

I'm not saying that an obese person is unhappy about being fat – some live with it quite well – but a person becomes fat when trying to offset a lack of well-being, dissatisfaction that can vary according to how easily frustrated they get, or vulnerability when dealing with hardships and difficulties in their life. Even if this is not an easy thing to hear, it is the truth. And there's never any lack of respect in this; quite the opposite. Denying problems has never resolved them – not for the patient, or for the doctor. And I keep saying this: people don't choose to grow fat, nobody wants to become fat. No nutritionist worthy of the name would say anything different. And many psychologists will confirm it. Whenever food becomes an addiction, there's always some subconscious reason for it. Whatever it is, addiction conceals a hidden misery, which an empathetic doctor like me cannot ignore and feels compelled to alleviate – hence my 'ten pillars of happiness'. To say that being overweight is simply down to recipes and calories and that to lose weight we need only eat less and be more active just isn't enough – and it doesn't work. It's a very officious way of acting as if something was actually being done to help people lose weight, an indirect way of backtracking and telling people to carry on being fat. I cannot possibly go along with this sort of attitude, which I deem to be irresponsible.

Sugar = The Enemy

If my first front's worldwide success has earned me much criticism, I'm pleased to see that today I'm not the only one fighting against sugar. This is what I'm going to explain to you now. Throughout the book I've talked about sugar at length, describing how harmful it is for you. For me, sugar is our number one public enemy. However, once again, let's examine the facts together – I'm keen to give you the information to gain your support, by providing evidence.

First of all, our dietary allowance.

In 1950, the FAO (Food and Agriculture Organization for the United Nations), established in 1945 and funded mostly by the United States, decreed that the dietary allowance for a person in the West should include 55–60 per cent carbs, fast and slow sugars included.

Why? When so many different dietary models were available across the world, what was this recommendation based on and where did the consensus for it come from? There isn't really an answer.

And, more than 60 years on, how is it conceivable that these standards, which are coming increasingly under

attack, still remain in force? Our lifestyle has become sedentary. And yet a sedentary person scarcely uses any more
calories than a paraplegic. Anyone could straightaway see
that dietary allowances ought to be modified to match the
level of physical activity. This is plain common sense. And
yet we carry on undeterred, told to eat the same amount of
carbs as before. Carbs are used to provide energy – but with
our sedentary, urban, mechanized lives we need far fewer.
Strange? Not as strange as you may think.

That the FAO, which provides a framework for the
food-processing sectors, should promote a recommendation of this kind was understandable, even logical. But
that the scientific *establishment* continues to defend its
application reveals the close ties, not to say the collusion,
between these various players in society. Let's suppose
that innocence prevails and that no converging interests
exist. A theoretical position of this kind should still be
questioned and revised in light of the alarming worldwide weight statistics. As far as scientific ethics go, this
would be the bare minimum. Any medical approach
involves sticking to the actual facts, describing symp-
toms, finding causes and providing treatment.

As long as a country's proportion of GDP that makes
money out of weight problems is greater than the health
bills for tackling weight diseases, nobody is really going
to do battle. This is what I think, what I've told you and it
makes me very angry. Even if, each year, proactive talk
and protests are heard from the country's health and
political bodies, in reality nothing decisive and effective

happens afterwards. What's worse, these flawed recommendations continue to be made, thereby ensuring profits for the food-processing sectors and indirect profits for much of the pharmaceutical industry, which grows rich from the damage caused by weight problems and obesity. The status quo holds sway and public health sees no gain, to say the very least.

A wide scientific and humanist school of thought also believes that sugar and fast carbs are not human foods and that it's dangerous to have too much. Here are two of the most high-profile examples.

Professor Robert Lustig has been leading the fight in America. A professor of pediatrics, he is Director of the Weight Assessment for Teen and Child Health (WATCH) Program at the University of California in San Francisco. Working on this public mission, he became alarmed and outraged that 17 per cent of American children and teenagers are obese.

According to the American Heart Association, the average adult consumes 22 teaspoons of sugar per day and teenagers as many as 34 teaspoons!

In 2012, he published a study in the prestigious journal *Nature*, which shook American public opinion. In it he stated that sugar, and especially fructose, presents such enormous risks for public health that it should be seen as a substance needing regulation in the same way as alcohol or tobacco. Over the past 50 years, worldwide sugar consumption has tripled. This upsurge has helped create a global obesity pandemic that causes 35 million deaths across the world through different illnesses, notably diabetes, cardiac diseases and cancer.

To try to halt this consumption, Professor Lustig recommends taxing sugary foods and regulating sales to children under the age of 17: 'We need worldwide regulation to reduce sugar consumption as there's no medication capable of intervening. All the doctors and researchers who've worked on it know this. We've investigated and examined all the pathways the body uses to metabolize sugars, searching for a possible element or space to develop a molecule that could intervene and there's no possibility. All we can do is cut down our intake.'

Professor Lustig clearly states that our physiology cannot deal with an excessive influx of sugars and that we have to REDUCE our daily amount. This is precisely what I've been telling you.

Another voice has been raised in the fight against weight problems and obesity, a very important voice that spoke out with great courage and lucidity.

On 11 September 2012 at a meeting on the island of Malta, **Dr Margaret Chan, Director-General of WHO**, gave a speech to European health ministers at the Regional Committee for Europe. It was an exceptionally bold warning.

She is outraged by the role of the food industry lobbies in the weight epidemic and is campaigning for the production of sugary snack foods to be regulated. Rather than comment on her address, I prefer to give you the most important sections from the speech:

Today, the struggle to safeguard public health increasingly places health concerns in competition with the interests of powerful multinational corporations. Any health policy, no matter how sound or far-sighted, that is perceived to threaten a fragile economy risks being put aside in the drive for economic growth and a strong GNP (gross national product).

For example, the best way for populations to lose weight is for the food industry to sell less unhealthy food, especially food that is cheap, convenient and tasty, but energy rich and nutrient poor. For obvious reasons, this will never happen all by itself.

Industrialized, highly processed food is becoming the new dietary staple around the world in what some researchers call the 'snack attack'.

Marketing budgets are big and audiences very well targeted. Links to the prevalence of obesity and related diseases are well documented. As with tobacco control, reversing this trend depends on support from policies in multiple non-health sectors.

Many of the concepts addressed in your documents have their roots in this Region. I find it entirely appropriate for Europe to continue its leadership role by giving these concepts a concrete body of evidence, supported by a diversified menu of policy options . . .

Again, think about obesity, especially childhood obesity, and the clever marketing of unhealthy foods and beverages to children, beamed by satellite

385

TV . . . Our world is in bad trouble. Multiple troubles have multiple consequences for health . . .

As I have said before, health is on the receiving end of policies made in other sectors. I have no illusions. Likewise, we understand the daunting challenges for you as ministers of health. Within governments and internationally, the health sector will never have as much power, or as many resources, as sectors like finance, trade or defence.

This likely reflects the tendency of political leaders to define a very narrow national progress agenda, as measured by economic growth and a rising GNP.

'Snack attack', 'energy rich, cheap but unhealthy foods' and the power of the food manufacturers' lobbies – what I've been denouncing year after year – have been publicly denounced, and to the whole planet, by a WHO official. The message is clear, to the point and final. Like me, WHO advocates solutions to do away with processed products containing too many calories, too much sugar and too much flour.

However, nutritionists are still divided about allocating responsibility respectively to the three universal nutrients – carbs, fats (lipids) and proteins – for the great non-infectious pandemics: obesity, diabetes, cardiovascular diseases, cancer and Alzheimer's disease.

With regard to **diabetes**, sugars are included in the actual definition of the disease; a person becomes diabetic once the level of sugar in 1 litre of blood exceeds 1.26g.

As for **cardiovascular diseases**, which often occur with diabetes, responsibility is now shifting away from fats and even cholesterol towards sugar, as we learn more about its pernicious effect on the arteries.

When it comes to **obesity**, for fear of being forced to abandon the dogma that all calories are equal, there is refusal to accept that insulin is lipogenic and creates weight problems.

As for **cancer**: ketogenic (very low carb) diets now form part of the treatment; reducing the cancer's virulence and proliferation of metastases. A normal cell functions with all fuels (glucose, fatty acids and ketones produced from proteins). If there's no glucose in the blood, the cancerous cell is no longer able to feed itself, so it stops multiplying. What more is there to say?

Finally, with regard to **Alzheimer's disease**, diabetologists all maintain that diabetes is the primary nutritional risk factor for this disease.

Sugar is by far the most dangerous nutrient there is for humans. We aren't equipped with the necessary organs to eat it without risk. For millennia our species lived very well without sugar; it's only since the nineteenth century that sugar has been produced industrially through sugarbeet extraction.

As for fat, our natural food reserve, we needed it to cope with and survive food shortages. Nowadays, we're coping with the exact opposite: an overabundance of food supplies.

However, sugar is far, far more dangerous than fat because the calories in sugar are much more dangerous and fattening than others. For more than 40 years this is what I've seen time and again, and seen confirmed time and again. Fortunately, mindsets are changing, which pleases me greatly.

The Culmination Of My Career: The ObÉpi Study

Hostile coalitions, criticism and opposition are now an everyday part of my life and my fight to stop you being overweight. However, amid this turmoil, I was waiting for the moment of truth, when the results of the ObÉpi France study would be published. The ObÉpi France study is a regular periodic census of the overweight population in France.

ObÉpi-Roche is an institution that carries out a national survey, whose authority is universally acknowledged. It aims to record the prevalence of weight problems and obesity across France. It combines different criteria (age, gender, weight, BMI, waist size, region, income, etc.) to ensure that its statistics are as realistic as possible.

It has been carrying out research for the past 15 years and publishes a report every three years.

Here are the percentages showing the increase in obesity over 15 years:

8.5% in 1997
10.1% in 2000

11.9% in 2003
13.1% in 2006
14.5% in 2009
15.0% in 2012

Over the first 12 years, from 1997 to 2009, ObÉpi recorded a 6% increase in obesity, with an average increase of 1.5% every three years.

With a sudden halt in this upsurge, its latest publication covering the 2009 to 2012 period shows, for the first time in its history, a very clear slowdown: dropping from 1.4% to just **0.5% over three years** (i.e. almost three times less).

Specifically, this 0.5% means that **during this period, 458,420 French people managed to avoid obesity, and the diseases and complications that come with it, and were no longer condemned to live nine years less than others**.

The study also quantified the increase in related risks due to obesity:

• *High blood pressure*

The obese are treated 3.6 times more often for high blood pressure than others.

In 2009, 18.4% of the population said it was being treated for high blood pressure and 17.6% in 2012, i.e. a 0.8% decrease. This means that 360,000 people have stopped high blood pressure treatment because they no longer need it.

• *Dyslipidemia, cholesterol and triglycerides*

Another lesson from this study: the obese are treated 2.7 times more often for their cholesterol and triglycerides than others.

• *Type 2 diabetes*

In France there are 7 times more diabetics treated among the obese than in other groups.

• *Cardiovascular risk*

The combination of the three major risks of diabetes, cholesterol and high blood pressure is 14 times higher for the obese.

How can I see these results as the crowning achievement of my medical career? Because the period in question (2009–2012) coincides with the publication of my diet and it's my firm belief that I helped achieve this result. However, I prefer to remain objective and analyze the facts covering these three years.

Three independent studies establish my method's ranking from 2009 to 2012:
1. In 2011, the French market research institute **TNS Sofres**, without even telling me, listed the top five of the 15 most commonly used weight-loss diets in France as:

- The Dukan method (30%)
- The Weight Watchers diet (11%)
- The Cabbage Soup diet (9%)
- Dr Cohen's method (4%)
- Dr Delabos' Chrononutrition diet (2%)

2. In 2012, the same institute carried out the same survey, with an improved percentage as Dukan method users had jumped from 30% to 36%.

3. The **NutriNet-Santé** study. This is one of the most important epidemiological studies in the world for eating behaviour and the relationship between nutrition and health. It was launched on 11 May 2009 and directly monitors a population of 500,000 participants (nutrinautes). Controlled by **INSERM** (French National Institute of Health and Medical Research) and by many research bodies and universities, supported by the French Ministry of Health, the French National Institute for Prevention and Health Education, the French Institute for Public Health Surveillance and Foundation for Medical Research, it is serious and independent.

What does this study say?

'Two-thirds of nutrinautes – 66% – who followed a diet supported by a method followed the Dukan method.'

This is the breakdown for all the nutrinautes who were dieting:

Dukan	66.1%
Cohen	11.2%

Chrono	11%
Montignac	3.7%
Cabbage Soup	2.9%

When asked about ease of use: 62% of those following the Dukan Diet found it easy; 12.4% found it difficult; 25% found it neither difficult nor easy.

As for long-term weight stabilization: 51.4% (i.e. the majority of users) considered that the Dukan Diet 'worked over the long term'.

On the one hand, the ObÉpi study results show that between 2009 and 2012 a novel phenomenon happened: a marked slowdown in obesity. One expert, Dr M.-A. Charles, said this about the figures: 'The ObÉpi study cannot shed light on the cause or more likely the causes for this slowdown.'

On the other hand, during this same period, three different studies, two carried out by the TNS Sofres Institute in 2011 and 2012 and the NutriNet study, all show that during the years when this marked slowdown took place, it was my diet that most French people were following.

What other factor could have appeared on the diet or method scene that could help explain this phenomenon, which is anything but trivial since it lifted half a million obese people out of the French obesity statistics?

As far as I know, no new weight-loss method or medication appeared in France during this time.

As for the French **National Nutrition and Health Programme (PNNS)** campaigns, they're important because they establish nutritional guidelines that promote certain categories of food and drink while recommending that others are limited. This means that they are more concerned with preventing weight problems than fighting the scourge. These campaigns have been around since 2001 and were extended in 2006 and 2011.

I draw the logical conclusion that a clear and significant blow has been dealt to the worrying increase in weight problems in France, during a period when my method was the one most widely used. I'm not claiming exclusive credit for this, but that I made a contribution seems to me indisputable.

Conclusion

As you close this book, you know that my method has been split in two and has an additional front. You can now decide which front is best suited to your own temperament, personality and weight background.

The first front is demanding, but rapid, powerful and motivating. Choice is limited but quantities are not. It's structured, prescriptive, allows no room for hunger, requires commitment but is wonderfully suitable for anyone whose motivation feeds off the joy of losing weight. Alongside this first front, a second front has been opened. This one I devised for people who are less hung up about their weight, in less of a hurry, less motivated by an underlying health risk and who wish from the very first week of dieting to continue enjoying a really wide range of foods.

I've painted a portrait of both profiles but now it's up to you to choose. Go where your temperament and mood take you. I can guarantee you that whichever front you select for tackling your weight problems, if you follow your road map as I suggest to you, you'll start losing weight and then you'll stabilize.

If you're equally torn between both profiles and can't decide which one to go for, visit my website **www. regimedukan.com**, answer the questions I give you and you'll find out which method is most suitable for you (like working out your True Weight, this service is free).

You probably bought this book because you hope to lose weight. It's clear that I've endeavoured to raise the debate by placing weight problems in their true context – that of human beings as we've always been, now struggling to cope not only with today's society but with tomorrow's, which already awaits us. Please believe that I'm not straying away from the topic. Quite the opposite: this is getting right to the heart of the matter. It's not generalizing but looking at specifics, at you specifically and your happiness, which is under threat.

Putting on weight isn't an illness; it's proof of being determined to survive humanly in an environment that makes this difficult.

Putting on weight indicates difficulties in finding fulfilment and searching for natural ways to counterbalance this dissatisfaction.

Since the human race started growing fat from 1944 onwards, and because our genes and physiology haven't changed, the reasons for us becoming overweight must lie in the way our lifestyle, society and civilization have evolved.

Whenever I'm talking to one of my overweight patients, I find myself confronted by two individuals inside the same person. The first one is invisible and doesn't speak; it's revealing behaviour patterns that give it away. What it wants is quite clear: it simply aspires to live and to get as much possible genuine pleasure, directly and without restriction. It isn't programmed to cater for you wanting to lose weight deliberately. Its role is to look after and protect your survival reserves. There's something animal in it, common to all mammals.

And then there's the other individual, the human who talks, expresses itself, thinks it's the only one around and believes itself capable of making decisions. It wants to lose weight, believing that all that's needed to sort the problem out is some technique or pill.

Nature or the evolution of the species has left nothing to chance or to the mercy of its most complex and sublime creature. Consciousness, reason and human intelligence are splendid tools, of course, and capable of improving what we do and how we control our world. But nature is cautious, and hasn't given us the right to take control of our life and protect it. We humans have assumed the right to control and exploit nature and, in so doing, to endanger it. But as for our own survival, eating and procurement of pleasure, all this remains under the absolute control of automatic physiological reflexes which, by definition, are totally dispassionate.

This is the reason why it has become so easy to put on weight nowadays, as we're all programmed to be unable to resist the need to eat and enjoy the food that makes us fat. And why it's so difficult not to put weight back on because our hold on life, our desire and need to stay alive are all subject to getting a dose of serotonin. And we have ten sources that can supply this vital fuel. But getting access to them is dependent on society's interests and bound up with our own childhood and background.

If you can grasp these ideas and make use of them, you'll lose weight far more easily and be far better placed to keep it off.

In this book, as well as introducing a new front for widening the fight against weight problems, I wanted you to gain insight into the area of your weight problems that's to do with your psychology, emotions, instincts and feelings.

I'm offering you both fronts as two infallible techniques for losing weight based on your profile, but only provided this is what you truly want.

'But of course it's what I want,' you'll tell me.

This isn't enough. You also need that part of you which doesn't speak to want it and to decide it too – this is really important.

This silent decision-maker is the animal, instinctual part, the biological controller that watches over you with robot consistency when you sleep and especially when you dream. Without its consent, you'll lose weight miserably and with difficulty. Perhaps you'll get down to your target weight but the robot will drive you to put the pounds you lose back on again.

To get your instinctual decision-maker's consent, you need to know how it operates. This is why I've laid such great stress on the overall context of being overweight, which lies somewhere between biological programming and the societal dimension, this antagonism between what your body seeks and what your society wants.

If you've put on weight, it's because you misunderstood the biological and cerebral rules about pleasure and your will to live. Study closely what you now know about serotonin and creating pleasure, about the pulsar and the will to live, about reward-seeking behaviour patterns, the ten pillars of happiness and the rule of swapping pleasures which works on the principle of symbiosis. And look at what our consumer society offers and learn to pick out what's compatible with what you want from life. Basically, learn to remain human while living in a society that is distancing itself from our deeper nature.

As I'm about to leave you, I'd like to make a wish, which is that I've helped you. Most likely we'll never have the opportunity to meet, but remember that I wrote this book with the sole purpose of giving you my most caring and competent advice. I do this out of pure gratitude because my readers – and now you're one of them – have given me such an immense amount. I've chalked up much experience, and as many years, so that each time I write a book I always wonder – it's a ritual – if I'll be here to write the next one.

Of the books I've written, I consider this one to have the most hope of changing things. It joins my first book,

The Dukan Diet, offering an alternative to it and enabling my work to reach a wider public.

Don't forget that if you have something important to ask me or tell me, here is my personal email address: docteurpierredukan@gmail.com

Index

401

Index

Index

403

Index

Index

Index

Index

peppers
  tuna Provençal recipes 214–15
  vegetable tartare with chopped smoked
    salmon 174–5
pesticides in fruit 184–5
pharmaceutical industry 383
physical activity 27, 36, 37, 40, 64
  and the brain 186–7
  and energy 306
  giving up lifts and escalators 345–8
  need for 63–5
  and the Nutritional Staircase 136,
    164–5, 188, 209–10, 229, 251–2,
    271–2
  and sedentary lifestyles 382
  and serotonin 63–4, 164–5, 209, 345
  and Stabilization 339–40, 342–8
  and thermogenesis 132
  using the stairs 328
  see also walking
pigeon 109
pissaladière slices 213–14
pizza 208
  Dukan Neapolitan pizza 175–6
play, need for 60–1
pleasure
  and primitive man 44
  and the pulsar 47–8
  and serotonin 47, 54–5
porcini mushroom velouté 168–9
potatoes 240–1, 243
  baked 249
  Dukan-style raclette 263–4
  mashed 249
poultry 109
prawns
  sautéed Mediterranean prawns with
    caramelized ginger 146–7
pregnancy
  and True Weight 315
primitive man see hunter-gatherers
proteins
  and amino acids 201–2
  in cereals 202
  digesting 29, 131
  and the Dukan method 32–3
  first front 25, 25–6, 36, 37, 40,
    365–6
  and the kidneys 375–6
  protein Thursdays 40, 41, 324
    Stabilization 337–42, 348, 353, 354
  in ready meals 162–3

second front 105–16
  Consolidation phase 316, 317–18
  and thermogenics 131, 375
  vegetable proteins 111–16, 202–3
  as vital foods 201–3
the pulsar
  and pleasure 47–8
  and serotonin 53, 164–5

quails 109
quark 117
  cocoa ice cream with fresh raspberries
    198–9
  crusty, spicy turkey strips 145–6
  extra-light strawberry mousse 196–7
  quinoa and bresaola timbales 259–60
  vanilla cheesecake with raspberry coulis
    193–4
quinoa 245, 249–50
  double salmon tartare with red quinoa
    257–8
  quinoa and bresaola timbales 259–60

rabbit 105
raclette, Dukan-style 263–4
raspberries
  apple, pear and raspberry crumble
    195–6
  cocoa ice cream with fresh raspberries
    198–9
  vanilla cheesecake with raspberry coulis
    193–4
ready meals 161–3
rebound phenomenon 302–3, 370–1
  controlling 304–9
recipes
  Friday 231–8
  Monday 143–51
  Saturday 254–64
  Sunday 277–83
  Thursday 212–20
  Tuesday 168–77
  Wednesday 189–99
restaurant eating on Mondays 139–40
reward-seeking behaviour patterns 47,
    52–4
  and serotonin 73–4
rhubarb 155, 182
  rhubarb meringue compote 176–7
rice
  brown 248
  chicken liver risotto 254–5

Index

Index